Transformational Health Communication

Olaf Werder
Department of Media & Communications
The University of Sydney
Sydney, NSW, Australia

ISBN 978-981-99-9605-6 ISBN 978-981-99-9606-3 (eBook)
https://doi.org/10.1007/978-981-99-9606-3

Cover illustration: Brain light / Alamy Stock Photo

This Palgrave Macmillan imprint is published by the registered company Springer Nature Singapore Pte Ltd.
The registered company address is: 152 Beach Road, #21-01/04 Gateway East, Singapore 189721, Singapore

Paper in this product is recyclable.

Olaf Werder

Transformational Health Communication

A New Perspective on Healthcare and Prevention

palgrave
macmillan

To William

Preface

The beginning of my motivation to look deeper into health communication and its practice probably came when I wasn't even thinking about being an academic. In my last professional job in advertising before switching careers, my agency got involved with an organisation whose mission was to improve the lives of children, youth, and families facing significant health challenges or social isolation. To witness this not-for-profit's struggles and passion (including dealing with the stress of dealing with their clients' stigmatisation reactions) and to be able to use our skills for a worthy cause were rewarding to me. But it also gave me an initial glimpse into the wider implications of health, or rather its absence.

Years later, as a young academic researcher in strategic communication, I got involved with a childhood obesity effort that purposefully wanted to include the targeted audience in the planning and preparation of whatever the final output would look like. The enthusiasm with which the kids and some of their parents threw themselves behind this effort, and coming up with novel ideas, showed me how much people—if given the opportunity—are willing to work on their own and their community's health.

The revelations from these two occasions form the parentheses of sort of this book. As a trained and educated commercial persuasion scholar and professional, I probably brought a somewhat different understanding to the issues of audience response assessment, values propositioning in messages, win/loss frame weighting, and sender influence in health communication already. But those and other anecdotes related to the social implications of health, the often-uneasy relationship health promoters have with their target communities, the persistent concerns of inequality, to name a few, made me rethink how I position myself toward the structure, strategy, and process of my discipline.

I spent the past two decades exploring the applicability of a more humanistic angle to health marketing, promotion, and policy efforts, paying attention to the benefit of community involvement wherever possible. Hereby I had the fortune to work with a variety of scholarly as well as professional experts in health communication agencies, governments, multidisciplinary research institutes, not-for-profits, and non-government organisations, who have enriched my work and provided new insights into feasibilities, barriers, and possible directions. I trust that this book will also assist them and individuals and teams like them in their own endeavours.

As a former advertising professional, I am not only aware of but have been part of the power of good wordsmithing and strategic communication when trying to elicit a desired reaction or behaviour. In public health, this would pertain to improving the public's health status and promote behavioural change. As such, I am thankful and a big cheerleader to everyone who has gotten involved in providing these instructions to improve health campaigns.

I have come to realise though that the advancement of health, let alone the connected ideas of social equity and citizen (or health consumer) empowerment cannot be met by another tactical improvement in message design and delivery channel selection. The impasses and systemic cracks we have seen across the world during the height of the global COVID pandemic are illustrative of how much health is connected to other areas, such as politics and policymaking, science and education, and economics.

As such, we ought to rethink our approach to health communication and care on a more holistic level and transform it by making full use of its interdisciplinary nature, drawing more from disciplines as diverse as medical ethics, marketing, sociology, education, psychology, economics, public affairs, and the arts and humanities. This book was the result of my thoughts on how this may be possible, contributing to the ongoing discussions on this matter. Its ultimate purpose, of course, is to help train a new generation of health communicators who are comfortable with and embrace its ideas.

Sydney, NSW, Australia Olaf Werder

Declaration of Interests

The author declares that he has no known competing financial interests or personal relationships that could have appeared to influence the work reported in this book.

Acknowledgements

Several colleagues, friends, and family members have helped making this book what it has become in the end. My first thanks go to my editor, Marion Duval of Palgrave, for her guidance and patience in moving this book along.

Thanks also must go to the anonymous reviewers for their queries and suggestions that have made their way into the relevant chapters. I am also indebted to professional friends who have over the past months either provided ideas and feedback on early concepts and drafts or provided motivation when energy was low due to other heavy workloads. Among them are Kate Holland, Susan Thomas, Michael Hinner, Jaemin Jung, and Ian Maxwell. I am also very grateful to Theaanna Kiaos and Jay Munro, two of my former graduate students, who worked as a research assistant on some of my projects. The results, their dedicated work produced, have been instrumental to arrive at my thinking on some of the topics of this book. I am finally thankful to the many doctoral and post-graduate students who have informed this book via in-class and personal discussions on health communication.

I am convinced that without the numerous professionals and lay public partners, I had the good fortune to engage with, conduct research with, or exchange ideas and concerns with, this book would not have become what it has. Besides the invaluable contribution of these brainstorming sessions, it has sharpened and altered my thinking about the problems we still face in reaching people, i.e., how much we still need to learn.

Finally, my deep thanks go to my family, my wife Amy, for her support and partnership when I disappeared into the home office, and my baby boy, William, whose unbridled love of life has inspired me in many ways in this process. And to my mother, Erika Werder, who had softly but determinedly encouraged me for some time to "get it done" as only mothers can while struggling herself with health issues. Her dedication and love helped me to complete this book.

Contents

About the Author

Olaf Werder is a senior lecturer in the Faculty of Arts and Social Sciences at the University of Sydney, Australia, where he teaches courses and directs the postgraduate programme in health communication.

After a ten-year professional career in the communication industry in Germany and the United States, working in advertising and promotions, he held academic appointments at the University of Florida and the University of New Mexico in the United States prior to coming to Sydney.

Werder's fields of expertise include persuasive communication, health communication and identity, group/organisational communication in healthcare/promotion settings, and the connections of health communication to health humanities and social practice theories. Werder has authored several publications in his research interests and maintains an active research profile in looking for avenues to transform contemporary health communication into an exchange tool for ideas, meanings, and best practices that become a motivating force for behavioural change.

1

The Field of Health Communication: An Overview

Introduction

In 1998, Kreps and colleagues published what was regarded among the first textbook and concise historical abstract of the field of health communication. At that time, the field already looked back at a 25-year study of human and mediated communication in healthcare delivery and health promotion, mostly driven by scholars in North America at the time. Unsurprisingly, it was a US-based communication association that led to a greater academic institutionalisation when in 1973 the International Communication Association established the Therapeutic Communication Interest Group. The group then voted to rename itself in 1975 as the *Health Communication* Division. Between the mid-1980-and 1990s, other communication and public health associations followed in creating health communication groups, again spearheaded by associations in the United States, as were the creation of the first undergraduate and (post) graduate health communication majors. Altogether, by the late 1990s into the early 2000s, health communication as a research and teaching area had been firmly established.

O. Werder, *Transformational Health Communication*,
https://doi.org/10.1007/978-981-99-9606-3_1

But what precisely is health communication? As a starting point we may adopt Schiavo's (2007) definition as "*a multifaceted and -disciplinary approach to improve health outcomes via information sharing and education that serves to modify behaviours.*" In one way or another, this general idea has been largely adopted by many public health entities. The Centres for Disease Control and Prevention (CDC) (2011), for instance, defines health communication as "[t]he study and use of communication strategies to inform and influence individual decisions that enhance health." The U.S. Department for Health and Human Services (2010) calls it "the study and practice of communicating promotional health information, such as in public health campaigns, health education, and between doctor and patient." A 2009 Bulletin of the World Health Organization highlights its "emphasis on combining theory and practice in understanding communication processes for changing human behaviour" (Rimal & Lapinski, 2009). Finally, UNICEF (2015) describes its C4D (Communication for Development) approach—an area related to health communication focusing on developing countries—as "a systematic, planned and evidence-based strategic process, using a mix of communication tools, channels and consultative approaches to promote positive behavioural and social change."

In summary, health communication studies the role of human and mediated communication in achieving a health-related outcome. Ultimately, this outcome is the sustainability, improvement or enhancement of a targeted or general public's health. More directly, the outcome is a positive influence on future human behaviour to either change to a healthier or maintain a healthy lifestyle. Since communication can take many forms, such as interpersonal (dyadic or group), organisational (educational and corporate), cross-cultural, and mediated (traditional and digital media), this sub-discipline of studying communication about health logically deals with the same complexities as the larger field from which it is derived. While there is some consensus to group the discipline into communication for healthcare delivery, health promotion, risk communication, and, more recently, new information technologies (Kreps, 2009), health communication is by and large open to a host of theories, models, and strategies to examine phenomena but also debates and critiques about best approaches and precise objectives to achieve better health.

When one searches public health school's course and degree offerings of the major universities, let alone divisional or themed project activities of the world's major public health associations, one unavoidably finds the term 'health promotion' more readily than 'health communication.' It begs the question whether these terms are interchangeably used, or whether health communication is basically health promotion/community and public health (with health education added) by another name.

I admit that health promotion itself is a broad term that in its main objective to prevent causes of ill health encompasses a mix of "educational, economic, political, and persuasive actions to enable individuals and communities to increase control over and improve their health" (Howat et al., 2003). But health promotion, like all promotion, focuses on the mission and strategies of those in charge of the promotional activity. In that it preserves a unidirectional focus and is at most interested in psychological features of the promotion's recipients (like attitudes, behavioural intentions, beliefs) that can be incorporated into messages to make promotional tasks effective. It usually excludes those groups as communicative collaborators or contributors.

Whereas health communication shares the communicative features and orientations with health promotion, its main function or justification for existence is more aligned with the broader field of risk communication in that communication is seen and studied as a dialogue. This follows the recognition that people usually come to their own decisions on impending risks or challenges despite the accuracy of assessed risk information they received. Since those typically involve a combination of heuristics, intuitions, cultural norms, and other idiosyncratic reasons for acting or not, a well-put together promotional campaign often still fails to make communication about the health risks effective.

Instead, successful communication of health-related information requires a deep understanding of people's decision-making processes, and designing communications needs to take these heuristics into account. Health communication, as such, is a much more inclusive term of human and social group thinking and discourse. It borrows knowledge and theories from diverse disciplines to truly understand human interaction in all its forms and the reasons for why and how it occurs. Today where public confidence and trust in traditional sources of health-related information has become quite low and can easily be outmatched by myths and misunderstanding (often promulgated through social media) health communication's vaster reach (over health promotion) can be seen to regain control over the discourse of health issues as targeted groups are looked at as partners in the communicative process.

The idea of transformational health communication, the title proposes, might seem grandiloquent to some but in the spirit of the etymological origin of the word 'transformational' (change in shape/form from Latin) this book argues for a more holistic perspective and internalisation of the discipline and act of communicating to arrive at a 'better' way of delivering health messages. This, in short, means for health communication entities to drastically change one's awareness and rationale whether this means achieving more trust by the targeted public, providing more transparency, or creating more personalised or participatory campaigns.

Attempting to use one's communicative efforts as a bridge between complex medical knowledge and lay community awareness or an exchange tool for ideas, meanings, and best practices has the benefit of communication in health to become a motivating force for behavioural changes. Even more relevant, due to communication being the connector for mutual understanding and respect it achieves its main purpose, namely a better quality of life for those the communication is aimed at.

What this book then is about is less a focus on the techniques of persuasive communication but more on trying to explain what communication in general is, how it connects with various fields of study and practice, and how it can be a tool for what health communication ought to truly be about: translation, connection, and meaning making.

The Complexity of Communication

Health communication encompasses a variety of spoken, written, and computer-mediated texts and processes (Harvey & Koteyko, 2013). As a subfield of communication studies, it is equally broad in including methods and ideas from fields as diverse as media studies, psychology, sociology, anthropology, informatics, education, and science (here: medicine, epidemiology, nursing). By and large, the field of communication explores on the one side, the symbols and channels of communication processes and, on the other side, the reception and effect of those on the recipients of such processes. It is telling that for many practitioners and researchers in public health, the notion of communication is reduced to its contribution in strategic, often mass-mediated, marketing. It is hence not surprising that many public health practitioners equate health communication with health promotion.

It is admittedly difficult to accurately describe what communication in health entails, especially since promoting ideas and desired behaviours obviously requires some form of communication as well. Health promotion, as such, can be construed as a communication subfield or discipline, whose aim it is to design messages that achieve a desired outcome, typically behavioural responses. Equating the whole of health communication with that is what Lee and Garvin (2003) critiqued as a reductionist interpretation that regards health communication as a linear, unidirectional, expert-driven flow of information to appeal to cognitive individualistic capabilities. In simpler terms, an expert provides convincing reasons to a target group, who then follows this sage advice.

As most practitioners in the field can attribute to, it isn't all that easy to get average people to change their behaviour via persuasive communication, especially if it requires to give up a desired one. Since individual behaviours are impacted by the social environment, in which individuals live, communication in all its forms impacts population-wide norms regarding healthy living, which in turn influences personal attitudes. In short, the idea of health is a societal value rather than a personal choice (Anderson & Nishtar, 2011) and communication plays a crucial role for community dialogue and active participation in mutual health maintenance or improvement.

While communication is among the 'younger' academic disciplines, the focus of its research is essentially primordial since the ability to communicate made human evolution possible. To distinguish it from the discipline of linguistics, the aim of communication studies is not language itself but the forms and ways of transmitting language (or unspoken thoughts and ideas) over distance and time for a purpose to a receiver.

The more scientific analysis of purposeful communication has its origins in rhetoric and public speaking skills of the ancient Greeks and Romans.

While rhetoric studies the art of perfecting persuasive oratory skills, the resolution disagreement through measured agreeable discussion, known as the dialectic method, played an equal role to the ancient Greeks and Romans. As such, there has always been a separation—some may call it a tension—between a focus on the original communicator and her reasons for communicating and skills to achieve her goals, on the one side, and a more relational function of communication among groups, on the other side. As we shall see, along the evolution of communication study, the former aspect has received more interest. Ironically, it is the latter idea of communication, the mutual solution finding, from which the root of the word itself stems. The word 'communication' comes from the Latin *communicare* (to share or to make common) and *communis* (belonging to all).

In the early twentieth century, writers, philosophers, and scholars (a growing number in the new field of journalism) still considered communication processes "a central and constitutive place in the study of social relations" (Cooley, 1909) or a force that "by itself creates a community" (Dewey, 1927). With the rise of electronic communication technologies and mass media after World War II the focus shifted onto a more scientific interest of how best to disseminate information. The rise of mass communication not only led to debates of the new role of the media in a democracy, famously summarised by Lippmann's (1922) critique of a "manufacture of consent," but the growing interest in the information processing capacity of communication led to the first theory of effective communication between a sender and a receiver.

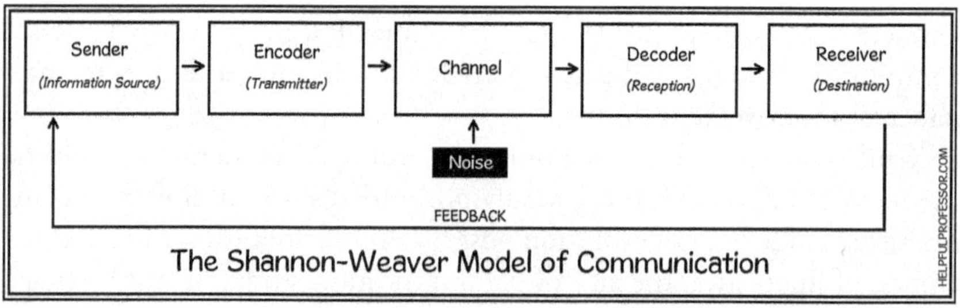

Source: Drew, C. (February 17, 2023). Shannon Weaver Model of Communication – 7 Key Concepts. Helpful Professor. https://helpfulprofessor.com/shannon-weaver-model/

Created in 1948 by American mathematicians Claude Shannon and Warren Weaver, it was officially called a "Mathematical Theory of Communication" (Shannon, 1948; Shannon & Weaver, 1949) but became known and popular among communication scholars as the "Shannon-Weaver model of communication" or "Communication Loop model." While it was originally meant to visualise the flow of electronic communication (the transfer of voice to electronic signals and back in a phone call), it was quickly adopted in the social sciences, especially communication science, as a model of models (Hollnagel & Woods, 2005) that explains in a simple way the communication process. While it has subsequently been criticised to "misrepresent the true nature of human communication" (Maras, 2000), it is fair to say that communication enquiry became detached from the earlier study of the art of debate and relationship building. In its stead, persuasion and media effects concepts moved centre stage. Those areas were regarded as useful especially for purposeful or strategic communication needed in political campaigning, marketing, and public relations. Those fields, not coincidentally, grew in importance around the same time.

Persuasion

Given that much of contemporary persuasive communication campaigns rely on elaborate consumer research, it is quite ironic that this modern technique goes back to the Greek affinity for rhetoric and elocution, defined as the art of using speech to convince. Unlike this training in public speaking so popular in ancient times, the modern concept of persuasion developed between the 1940s and 1950s, fuelled by an interest in understanding (and possibly improving) the effects of propaganda (e.g., Doob, 1948; Hovland et al., 1953; Lasswell, 1927). These studies eventually led to interests in exploring factors that influence the effectiveness of social communications, and with many of those early propaganda researchers hailing from the discipline of psychology, research quickly turned to micro-level analyses of individual motivations and actions, engaging in laboratory studies on attitudes, beliefs, fears, norm compliance, etc.

Whereas this title does not and cannot attempt to detail the vast field of persuasion theories, it suffices to say that persuasion and social influence theories have had a profound effect on not just commercial marketing but also the way social and health interventions are executed by those in charge of them. The original idea that attitudinal responses are basically shaped by positive or negative reinforcements or stimuli (Skinner, 1938) was refined over the next decades to include prior attitudes and experiences (Sherif & Sherif, 1967), desires for consistency in one's life and rationalisation of one's (aberrant) behaviour (Festinger, 1957; Heider, 1958; Osgood & Tannenbaum, 1955), the ability to resist persuasion via inoculation (McGuire, 1961), and drives to make decisions free from influence (Brehm, 1966). I'll have more to say regarding resisting a persuasive health message in the next chapter.

Media Effects

Whereas media effects studies focus on the impact of all mediated communication on society, they have their origin in the analysis of the use of media for persuasion and propaganda. In addition, much of social (including health) promotion is largely conducted through some media channel so the interest of media effects research in behavioural science is equally relevant for mediated health promotion.

Media effects analysis started in the early twentieth century and has been subject to a spirited debate since then about how influential the media really are on people's opinion, attitude, or behaviour formation (Werder, 2009). Ultimately, media scholars never arrived at any unifying theory and still operate from perspectives on explaining the role of media in and on cultures and societies.

These different perspectives, in a nutshell, occupy the entire range from very powerful to very insignificant effects. On the one end are theories of powerful direct effects, known as hypodermic needle or magic bullet models, that assume that media messages are wholly accepted by a passive audience (Lasswell, 1948). It is noteworthy that this original "strong effects" theory is associated with the notion of a mechanical transmission model of direct effects linked to early theorists of information engineering (Neuman & Guggenheim, 2011), such as Claude Shannon, whose model I had outlined before (Shannon, 1948).

Next, we have models of subtle direct influences, whereby media exposure, over time, leads to certain perceptions of reality and—to use the name of the key theory—cultivate an audience's world view (Gerbner, 1970). Alternatively, the media's influence is not seen as direct but more circuitous. In one line of thought, media information flow is broken into two stages. That is, in the first stage, the mass media's effects are limited (or, shall we say, deliberately focused) on certain groups or individuals, known as opinion leaders. In the second stage, those become spokespersons to transmit the acquired mediated information to a wider population (Katz & Lazarsfeld, 1955). In another line of thought, the media do not control precisely what people think but they do control the topics what people think about. Known as agenda setting (McCombs & Shaw, 1972), this theory has taken a prominent place in media studies in terms of explaining the filtering or gatekeeping role of media. Finally, selectivity theories (Iyengar & Hahn, 2009; Klapper, 1960) and the uses and gratification models (Katz et al., 1973) take the opposite approach, assuming people are active not passive when consuming media, and choosing media content based on their own biases and desires or needs and hence media have a weak influence on attitudes and behaviours.

Communication in Health

What made health communication inquiry so exciting was its applied nature. For one, as a field within communication, it largely focuses on studying the influences of human communication on healthcare delivery and the promotion of public health. Unsurprisingly, one of its chief purposes is to directly apply findings and conclusions to the improvement of the quality of healthcare delivery and disease prevention (Smith, 1989). Consequently, besides being quite practically oriented, health communication inquiry is typically focused on certain problems in either health promotion or healthcare delivery. Those two perspectives typically determine whether the focus is on the persuasive use of communication messages and media to promote public health at large or on the way interpersonal and group communication influences the delivery of healthcare. That said, the distinction between those two has increasingly dissipated in the past years (Kreps et al., 1998).

For instance, despite healthcare delivery communication's ongoing emphasis on personal, direct discourse practices, such as doctor/patient communication and social support efforts, approaches more connected to health promotion (such as media channels) have seen a growing use via activities like telemedicine or online health education. At the same time, interpersonal or group-based efforts have been added to public health promotion (e.g., community prevention activities, corporate employee programmes, or government outreach efforts).

I do regard especially the latter as hopeful trends for a more participatory approach to prevention communication but am cognisant of the fact that the promotional wing of health communication has deep roots in psychological theories, which are usually unidirectionally oriented. As such, when discussing health promotional communication, especially that for non-communicable disease topics, similar—if not the same—patterns and debates regarding persuasion and media-borne effects that exist for the development of communication science in general apply to this niche.

Studying the properties of communication in health promotion in more depth, one often finds a heavy focus on the functional aspects of communication, i.e., the use of communication strategies and channels that follow model assumptions about the way people perceive, pay attention to, express, memorise, and think about specific health topics. Although the idea of communication as a mechanistic unidirectional flow of messages or signals over a medium to inform and influence individual decisions or responses existed since the late 1940s (see Shannon & Weaver, 1949), it was the arrival of the computer in the 1970s that impacted health promotion communication more profoundly by advancing the field of cognitive psychology. It was this field that due to its interest in information processing and delivery became interested in communication variables (Bandura, 1977; McGuire, 1984).

In a simplified way of expression, cognitive psychology rejected the idea of behaviourism that external stimuli drive behaviour and considered how mental processes influence behaviour more relevant to understand. The computer, thus, provided an apt terminology and metaphor to investigate information processing of the human mind (McLeod, 2015). As relevant as the linearity of cognitive processes akin to a computer analogy was the notion that human antecedents to behaviour can be studied by rigorous scientific laboratory methods. Whereas cognitive psychology has become relevant over the years for other fields (e.g., marketing, politics), it is unsurprising that it became rapidly attractive for the field of medicine, which itself operates from a mechanistic, science-driven, biomedical model of health.

Cognitive-behavioural theories, such as the Theory of Reasoned Action (Fishbein & Ajzen, 1975), the Health Belief Model (Janz & Becker, 1984; Rosenstock, 1974) or the Social Learning Theory (Bandura, 1977), suggest a mediational process (e.g., attention, beliefs, self-confidence, adherence to norms) between a stimulus and behavioural response. As the advancement of these theories coincided with the emerging literature in social marketing (Andreasen, 1994; Kotler & Zaltman, 1971; Rothschild, 1979), behaviour-oriented persuasive communication campaigns along the modelled paths became foundational elements for health promotions. Early prominent examples include the Stanford Heart Disease Prevention Program (Maccoby et al., 1985) and the North Karelia Project (Puska et al., 2016). What became a leading argument was that for a communicative intervention to be effective, it needs to understand what cognitive processes are predominant when a target person thinks about the health topic in question. Following that, a message that predominately speaks to that construct needs to be created.

For example, if people don't seem confident to follow a healthy diet due to lack of understanding what that means, then an obesity prevention campaign needs to focus on simple information, education, and encouragement. If, for the same issue, people highlight a need to fit in with others, then suggesting the existence of social norms related to slim bodies would be a driver. In general terms, if the content of a message can influence attitudes, beliefs, confidence levels, or whatever seems to be the leading variable to explain the current lack of behaviour towards a particular health (or rather lifestyle) condition, then the desired resulting behaviour would follow. It became evident that the effectiveness of such campaigns requires a broad understanding of not only underlying cognitive theories but procedural details of campaign development, including audience segmentation, mediated channel values, competition, and tactical executions. Hence, by the 1980s, health promotion started embracing social marketing, a field that borrows commercial marketing practices to achieve behavioural change within societies (Lefebvre & Flora, 1988).

The Growth of Social Marketing Approaches in Health Communication

Communication has always been a critical element in commercial marketing, fulfilling a central role in changing consumers' perception of a brand, product, or service, or motivating them to purchase or try it. Originally though communication had been equated with persuasion, which has rendered it a one-way process in transaction-based marketing strategies and executions. As I have shown above, communication theory has argued since the 1970s (e.g., Schramm, 1973) that persuasion is but one of many approaches in communication. The realisation of this integrative capacity of communication has led in the 1980s and 1990s to evolving theory shifts in marketing towards integrated and relationship models (Duncan & Moriarty, 1998). The importance of customer relationships has soon become accepted as one of the most important company assets, yet the move towards more relationship-based models has been more intuitive, lacking a deeper understanding of communication's role (Duncan & Moriarty, 1997; Grönroos, 1990).

Although social marketing has its own historic evolution, it is no surprise that at the same time that marketing moved towards a relationship-building model, the academic debate in social marketing shifted from the question "Should marketing be applied to social issues?" to the question "How can marketing be applied to social issues?" It was during those decades (1980s–1990s) that the health community began embracing the practice (MacFayden et al., 1999).

Health-related social marketing is usually defined as "the systematic application of marketing, alongside other concepts and techniques, to achieve specific behavioural goals, to improve health and reduce health inequalities" (French & Blair-Stevens, 2006). Applying concepts and techniques drawn from the commercial sector to promote changes in diverse socially important behaviours (Andreasen, 1995), social marketing has been embraced by the public health community as a framework of operation that is very beneficial "in promoting the procedure of individual's behaviour change to (a) reduce social problems or (b) remove barriers that prevent behaviour change" (Kotler & Zaltman, 1971).

On the one hand, the rapid growth and popularity of social marketing techniques in health stems from a ruthless effectiveness in commercial marketing that demands from programme planners to understand the problem to be addressed, the audience to be targeted, and the environment in which the programme will be applied. In short, effective programme planning is based on addressing target consumers' wants and needs.

On the other hand, its ascendancy derives from a growing recognition of the inadequacy of heretofore standard approaches, namely giving people information and urging them to be healthy. The irony hereby is that while social marketing was critiqued for commercialising the social purpose of healthcare and promotion, it was much more attuned to understanding people's rationales for their actions and therefore capable to suggest ideas how best to support them than previous approaches which seemed to sell health, or rather a better behaviour towards health.

Over time social marketing campaigns have led to various success stories in promoting healthy behaviours among citizens from the community or group to the individual level (Cabrita & Do Rosário Cabrita, 2014). Among those successes were

1. The U.S. Center for Disease Control and Prevention's 2002–2006 multiethnic physical activity media program for tweens, called ***VERB*** (Huhman et al., 2006).
2. The internationally recognised sun protection campaign from Australia and New Zealand, titled ***Slip-Slop-Slap*** that launched in the 1980s (Iannacone & Green, 2014).
3. The Truth Initiative's (formerly, the American Legacy Foundation) youth smoking prevention campaign, known as ***TRUTH***, which started in the late 1990s (e.g., Farrelly et al., 2002).

Social marketing has been proven to be particularly useful in promoting an individual's behaviour change to reduce social problems or removing barriers that prevent said behaviour change. In so doing, it has been effective in changing health behaviours for entire target populations. However, subtle distinctions made in marketing between population categories, by using psychographic data to understand motivations and barriers, have often been less evident, and less commonly translated into campaigns or programmes (NSMC, 2006).

With a body of research on perception and belief systems—foremost the field of social psychology (e.g., Kruglanski & Boyatzi, 2012; Restle et al., 1964)—having concluded that individuals will select and rely on information consistent with their basic ideas and social conditions, the idea of whether or not the recipient of a health behaviour change message is complying with it, seems to depend not so much on the factual accuracy and persuasive tone of the message but more on "the degree to which (…) a person can receive, evaluate, and act on relevant information received from the outside on its own intrinsic merits" (Black, 2001; Rokeach, 1960).

Undeniably, social marketing contributed to a shift in health communication from a top-down quasi-mandatory solicitation of behaviour change to a public-centric voluntary change persuasion. As Andreasen (2006) argued, "social marketing is not concerned with changing held ideas and convictions but influencing behaviours." Yet, the imperfection in translating commercial thinking into this area of social welfare lies in an uneasy translation of the exchange of values between the parties.

While the public health community, or at the least, those who have embraced and operate with a social or health marketing framework, have come to understand the contributions of commercial marketing ideas of consumer-orientation, campaign planning, competition, audience segmentation, and evaluation, aspects of marketing tactics, such as the famous 4 P's (product, price, place, and promotion) and the exchange concept, remain difficult or elusive.

For instance, the mutual transmission of value seems an easy enough concept in the commercial sector. A consumer receives a product or service that s/he wanted and is hence willing to reimburse a vendor with its monetary equivalent. It is the so-called tit-for-tat idea and as ancient as barter trades. This idea is muddier when it comes to health behaviour modification. Offering an incentive for a voluntary behaviour change need to not only be something that a target person truly values but also be available around the same time so it can be 'exchanged.'

Conclusion

Health communication for behaviour change is a complex and challenging process as it is impacted both by internal attitudes and external structures. What people do in relationship to their health is in parts based on their knowledge, awareness, and/or beliefs about a lifestyle pattern they engage in. But it is equally a result of the communication of multiple (social) agents, even if those do not directly focus on health. Schramm's (1973) assessment about communication in general is equally relevant for the sub-discipline of health communication, namely that "to understand human communication we must understand how people relate to one another."

Consequently, human relationships are not possible without communication and thus health behaviours cannot be separated from political issues, economic and social circumstances, religious or cultural allegiances, societal norms, and the embedded interests of businesses, institutions, and professional groups (NSMC, 2006). Establishing 'behavioural goals' via health communicative efforts, therefore, requires going beyond the traditional focus on mediated behaviour change messages to recognise the dynamic nature of behaviour and relationships within a population.

One can appreciate that this causes some conceptual difficulties for creating lifestyle disease interventions (e.g., smoking, drinking, obesity) since the abandonment of a hedonistic pleasure to retain one's health in future decades seems a weak proposition for many people. An added complexity lies in the fact that aside from this perceived loss of a desirable behaviour, change is also associated with other intangible costs (e.g., time spent, psychic discomfort, etc.). And if this were not enough, if any intervention involves any intermediaries (e.g., doctors, digital content creators, associated health sector members), those groups must equally perceive a valued benefit in return for their contributions.

In the end, the overarching purpose of health communication is to identify people's own definition for their and their loved one's health and grasp and appreciate barriers and facilitators for their daily decisions and actions. While we often look for explanations for less effective campaigns in tactical or behaviour-theoretic reasons (wrong message, wrong media channels, wrong antecedent variable), the answer often lies in a lack of a shared understanding as a communication barrier. Using communication that is truly two-way or dialogical, i.e., lets the other side co-create meaning of current and future health conditions, is different from achieving transactional outcomes. Although this may seem like a semantic nuance, it lies at the heart of ongoing difficulties in achieving desired results in health promotion. Not being able to speak the same language or interpret responses to information correctly but making implicit assumptions that communication can be controlled (note that this goes back to the information processing model of communication) leads to distortions and misinterpretations of what needs to happen. Only engaging health message recipients in an honest dialogue can remedy this gap.

This title therefore aims to refocus the typical discussion in health communication by introducing a broader interdisciplinary approach when talking about communication. It expands beyond the usual health communication topics by including studies in social movements, concepts of agency, social representation theory, and constructions of critical public health paradigms. In so doing, it also aims to locate the scholarly debate of health communication as a dynamic process filtered by individual and social prisms that create complexity of health behaviour determinants, which in turn pose difficulties for interventions, and require a multidisciplinary approach for effectively communicating about health.

Overview of the Book

The book's chapters follow the tenets of the analytical process (Gale et al., 2013; Thomas, 2011), i.e., each of the earlier chapters serves to decompose the problem in health communication into relevant subproblems that find root causes for each subproblem, followed by the subsequent chapters providing explanation for issues raised and leverage points for potential resolutions.

Specifically, Part I presents three current barriers for more effective health communication. Part II offers reasons where these barriers and the lack of effective communication might come from. Finally, Part III suggests new thinking in approaching communicating health that takes the above barriers into account and provides ideas for reducing or eliminating them.

References

Anderson, P., & Nishtar, S. (2011). Communicating the non-communicable. *Journal of Health Communication: International Perspectives, 16*(s2), 6–12.
Andreasen, A. (1994). Social marketing: Its definition and domain. *Journal of Public Policy and Marketing, 13*(1), 108–114.
Andreasen, A. (1995). *Marketing social change: Changing behaviour to promote health, social development, and the environment.* Jossey-Bass.
Andreasen, A. (Ed.) (2006). *Social Marketing in the 21st Century.* Thousand Oaks, CA: Sage Publications. https://doi.org/10.4135/9781483329192.
Bandura, A. (1977). *Social learning theory.* Prentice Hall.
Black, J. (2001). Semantics and ethics of propaganda. *Journal of Mass Media Ethics, 16*(2), 121–137.
Brehm, J. (1966). *A theory of psychological reactance.* Academic Press.
Cabrita, M., & Do Rosário Cabrita, M. (2014). Applying social marketing to healthcare: Challenges and opportunities. In A. Kapoor & C. Kulshrestha (Eds.), *Dynamics of competitive advantage and consumer perception in social marketing* (1st ed., pp. 78–97). IGI Global.
Centers for Disease Control and Prevention. (2011). *Health communication basics.* http://www.cdc.gov/healthcommunication/healthbasics/whatishc.html
Cooley, C. (1909). *Social organization: A study of the larger mind.* Scribner.
Dewey, J. (1927). *The public and its problems.* Henry Holt & Co.
Doob, L. (1948). *Public opinion and propaganda.* Henry Holt & Co.
Duncan, T., & Moriarty, S. (1997). *Driving brand value: Using integrated marketing to drive stakeholder relationships.* McGraw-Hill.
Duncan, T., & Moriarty, S. (1998). A communication-based marketing model for managing relationships. *Journal of Marketing, 62*(2), 1–13.
Farrelly, M., Healton, C., Davis, K., Messeri, P., Hersey, J., & Haviland, M. (2002). Getting to the truth: Evaluating national tobacco countermarketing campaigns. *American Journal of Public Health, 92*(6), 901–907.

Festinger, L. (1957). *A theory of cognitive dissonance*. Stanford University Press.
Fishbein, M., & Ajzen, I. (1975). *Belief, attitude, intention and behavior: An introduction to theory and research*. Addison-Wesley.
French, J., & Blair-Stevens, C. (2006). *It's our health! Realizing the potential of effective social marketing*. National Social Marketing Centre.
Gale, N., Heath, G., Cameron, E., Rashid, S., & Redwood, S. (2013). Using the framework method for the analysis of qualitative data in multi-disciplinary health research. *BMC Medical Research Methodology, 13*, 117–124.
Gerbner, G. (1970). Cultural indicators: The case of violence in television dramas. *The Annals of the Academy of Political and Social Science, 388*, 69–81.
Grönroos, C. (1990). *Service management and marketing*. Lexington Books.
Harvey, K., & Koteyko, N. (2013). *Exploring health communication: Language in action*. Routledge.
Heider, F. (1958). *The psychology of interpersonal relations*. Wiley.
Hollnagel, E., & Woods, D. (2005). *Joint cognitive systems: Foundations of cognitive systems engineering*. Taylor & Francis.
Hovland, C., Janis, I., & Kelley, H. (1953). *Communication and persuasion: Psychological studies of opinion change*. Yale University Press.
Howat, P., Maycock, B., Cross, D., Collins, J., Jackson, L., Burns, S., & James, R. (2003). Towards a more unified definition of health promotion. *Health Promotion Journal of Australia, 14*(2), 82–85. https://doi.org/10.1071/HE03082
Huhman, M., Potter, L., Duke, J., Judkins, D., Heitzler, C., & Wong, F. (2006). Evaluation of a national physical activity intervention for children. *American Journal of Preventive Medicine, 32*(1), 38–43.
Iannacone, M., & Green, A. (2014). Towards skin cancer prevention and early detection: Evolution of skin cancer awareness campaigns in Australia. *Melanoma Management, 1*(1), 75–84.
Iyengar, S., & Hahn, K. (2009). Red media, blue media: Evidence of ideological selectivity in media use. *Journal of Communication, 59*, 19–39.
Janz, N., & Becker, M. (1984). The health belief model: A decade later. *Health Education Quarterly, 11*(1), 1–47.
Katz, E., Blumler, J., & Gurevitch, M. (1973). Uses and gratification research. *Public Opinion Quarterly, 37*, 509–523.
Katz, E., & Lazarsfeld, P. (1955). *Personal influence: The part played by people in the flow of communication*. Free Press.
Klapper, J. (1960). *The effects of mass communication*. The Free Press.
Kotler, P., & Zaltman, G. (1971). Social marketing: An approach to planned social change. *Journal of Marketing, 35*(3), 3–12.

Kreps, G. (2009). Health communication theories. In K. Foss & S. Littlejohn (Eds.), *Encyclopedia of communication theory* (pp. 464–469). Sage.

Kreps, G., Bonaguro, E., & Query, J., Jr. (1998). The history and development of the field of health communication. In L. Jackson & B. Duffy (Eds.), *Health communication research: Guide to developments and directions* (pp. 1–15). Greenwood Press.

Kruglanski, A., & Boyatzi, L. (2012). The psychology of closed and open mindedness, rationality, and democracy. *Critical Review, 24*, 217–232.

Lasswell, H. (1927). The theory of political propaganda. *American Political Science Review, 21*(3), 627–631.

Lasswell, H. (1948). The structure and function of communications in society. In L. Bryson (Ed.), *The communication of ideas* (pp. 37–51). Harper.

Lee, G., & Garvin, T. (2003). Moving from information transfer to information exchange in health and health care. *Social Science & Medicine, 56*, 449–464.

Lefebvre, R., & Flora, J. (1988). Social marketing and public health intervention. *Health Education Quarterly, 15*(3), 299–315.

Lippmann, W. (1922). *Public opinion*. Harcourt.

Maccoby, N., Farquhar, J., & Fortmann, S. (1985). The community studies of the Stanford heart disease prevention program. In R. Kaplan & M. Criqui (Eds.), *Behavioral epidemiology and disease prevention* (NATO ASI series (series a: Life sciences)) (Vol. 84, pp. 385–400). Springer.

MacFayden, L., Stead, M., & Hastings, G. (1999). A synopsis of social marketing. *Health Promotion International, 9*(1), 59–63.

Maras, S. (2000). Beyond the transmission model: Shannon, Weaver, and the critique of sender/message/receiver. *Australian Journal of Communication, 27*(3), 123–142.

McCombs, M., & Shaw, D. (1972). The agenda-setting function of mass media. *Public Opinion Quarterly, 36*(2), 176–187.

McGuire, W. (1961). Resistance to persuasion conferred by active and passive prior refutation of the same and alternative counterarguments. *Journal of Abnormal and Social Psychology, 63*, 326–332.

McGuire, W. (1984). Public communication as a strategy for inducing health promoting behavioral change. *Preventive Medicine, 13*(3), 299–319.

McLeod, S. (2015). *Cognitive psychology*. Retrieved August 21, 2022, from https://www.simplypsychology.org/cognitive.html

National Consumer Council. (2006). *It's our health!* National Social Marketing Centre.

Neuman, W., & Guggenheim, L. (2011). The evolution of media effects theory: A six-stage model of cumulative research. *Communication Theory, 21*, 169–196.
Osgood, C., & Tannenbaum, P. (1955). The principle of congruity in the prediction of attitude change. *Psychological Review, 62*(1), 42–55.
Puska, P., Basilal, S., & Narula, J. (Eds.). (2016). The North Karelia project. *Global Heart, 11*(2), 171–266.
Restle, F., Andrews, M., & Rokeach, M. (1964). Differences between open- and closed-minded subjects on learning-set and oddity problems. *The Journal of Abnormal and Social Psychology, 68*(6), 648–654.
Rimal, R., & Lapinski, M. (2009). Why health communication is important in public health. *Bulletin of the World Health Organization, 87*(4), 247.
Rokeach, M. (1960). *The open and closed mind: Investigations into the nature of belief systems and personality systems*. Basic Books.
Rosenstock, I. (1974). The health belief model and preventive health behaviour. *Health Education & Behavior, 2*(4), 354–386.
Rothschild, M. (1979). Marketing communications in non-business situations: Or, why it's so hard to sell brotherhood like soap. *Journal of Marketing, 43*(2), 11–20.
Schiavo, R. (2007). *Health communication: From theory to practice*. Wiley.
Schramm, W. (1973). *Men, messages, and media: A look at human communication*. Harper & Row.
Shannon, C. (1948). A mathematical theory of communication. *The Bell System Technical Journal, 27*(July and October), 379–423, 623–656.
Shannon, C., & Weaver, W. (1949). *The mathematical theory of communication*. University of Illinois Press.
Sherif, C., & Sherif, M. (Eds.). (1967). *Attitude, ego-involvement, and change*. Wiley.
Skinner, B. (1938). *The behavior of organisms: An experimental analysis*. Appleton-Century.
Smith, D. (1989). Studying health communication: An agenda for the future. *Health Communication, 1*(1), 17–27.
Thomas, G. (2011). A typology for the case study in social science following a review of definition, discourse, and structure. *Qualitative Inquiry, 17*(6), 511–521.
U.S. Department of Health and Human Services, Office of Disease Prevention and Health Promotion. (2010). *Healthy People* (Vols. 1 and 2, Chap. 11, pp. 11–20).

United Nations Children's Fund (UNICEF). (2015). *Communication for Development: Communication Lies at the Heart of Sustainable Development. C4D definition [Internet]*. UNICEF. https://www.unicef.org/cbsc/
Werder, O. (2009). Media effects theories. In K. Foss & S. Littlejohn (Eds.), *Encyclopedia of communication theory* (pp. 632–635). Sage.

Part I

Current Barriers to More Effective Health Communication

2

A Failure to Communicate

Overview

In the 1967 Paul Newman movie classic 'Cool Hand Luke,' Captain, the prison warden of Road Prison 36, utters the memorable movie line "*What we've got here is failure to communicate*" to justify beating the rebellious prisoner Luke Jackson played by Newman. He goes on saying: "Some men you just can't reach." I am reminded about this line every time another well-intended, researched, and strategically executed health promotion campaign fails to adequately reach the scores of people it was targeted at.

Clearly, it would be too simplistic to distil adverse results in antismoking, obesity prevention, and other comparable efforts to communication failure alone. Health inequalities, stigmatisation and unequal care of some groups, cultural discrepancies, and lack of comprehension of disease symptoms are but some of the factors that impact how we manage our health and hence interpret efforts to improve or maintain it. However, it is equally true that virtually all human knowledge is based on stories constructed around past experiences, and that new experiences are interpreted in terms of old stories (Howarth, 2011). As such, communicative

O. Werder, *Transformational Health Communication*,
https://doi.org/10.1007/978-981-99-9606-3_2

frames about health form a foundation for creating a system of common understanding, concepts, and ideas. Unfortunately, meanings associated with those frames often differ between various groups, such as different professional or lifestyle groups.

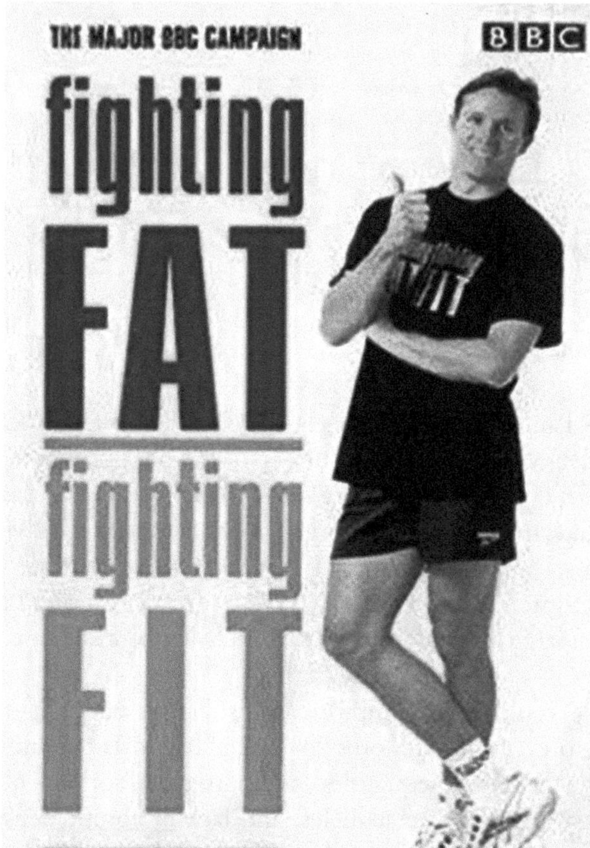

Let's use the following well-known and -researched late 1990s obesity prevention campaign in the UK, titled 'Fighting Fat, Fighting Fit' (or FFFF), as a classic example for the motivation or adoption issues we raise in this chapter. At the time, the FFFF campaign was the largest health education campaign ever undertaken by the country's largest broadcaster, the BBC. It comprised of a seven-week multi-media campaign, where target groups could call for further information, and ultimately register (at a nominal fee) to receive a self-help guide for lifestyle change as well as progress charts about their weight loss, activity levels, and eating habits (Wardle et al., 2001).

While this campaign admittedly relied basically on mass-media programming, it resulted in a common phenomenon of health promotion efforts. The FFFF campaign was very successful in getting its message in front of its target audience. In this case, about 62% had heard of the campaign. An equally sizeable number (about 34%) also recalled the campaign as being about healthy eating or increased physical activity, in short, understood its intent. However, those numbers did not reflect how many people agreed with it or acted upon it. In that respect, fewer than 1% actively participated. Although follow-up studies (e.g., Miles et al., 2001) pointed to the intricacies of obtaining accurate data, what appears to have happened was that this number was mainly comprised of normal-weight, active and higher socio-economic groups, who showed more sustained participation in the campaign than those most in need of lifestyle changes.

Lifestyles, Individuality, and Resistance

It would be silly to conclude from the term 'health resistance' that people wilfully resist health (lifestyle) interventions to achieve a different outcome than the one promoted akin to civil disobedience or related forms of economic or political non-cooperation. It is quite a complex concept, which has natural correlations to the cultural and social contexts of behaviour, as those contribute to the development of lifestyle choices. But it is precisely the turn towards affecting lifestyles (rather than addressing diseases) that makes discussing the issue of resistance timely and necessary.

In the 1970s, public health discourse shifted the way in which health promotion and illness prevention was approached by turning the focus towards lifestyle choices—such as smoking, alcohol, drugs, and dietary intake—and making the active preservation of good health and prevention of illness a responsibility of the individual (Briggs, 2003; Merrild et al., 2011).

An inherent dilemma for addressing lifestyle "problems" in this newly called "consumption of health" (Shilling, 2002) was that they do not simply exist in a values vacuum but are constructed in particular times and places by people with different viewpoints, living in particular socio-political environments (Bacchi, 1999). To say it in Williams' (1995) words: "*Health-related behaviour is a routinized feature of everyday life, (…) woven into its very fabric*" (p. 583).

Accordingly, the many health messages that come with "best practice" suggestions (do this, don't do that) can easily lead to a clash of viewpoints that may not only irritate or alienate the very groups that are targeted (Whitehead & Russell, 2004) but have also great potential to be perceived as paternalistic infringements by the message sender on one's autonomy (Eagle et al., 2003). To unravel the connection between those terms or effects more completely, we need to dive deeper into anthropological and sociological thoughts on the matter.

In 1980, Raymond Illsley published a study that asserted that people's general beliefs about health are a derivative of the degree to which people feel they have control over their daily lives. The latter, in turn, is shaped by their position within the broader social structure. A few years later, the medical sociologist, Michael Calnan published research that not only exposed the simple logic from knowledge to action as problematic but also showed how the average person's behaviour has its own logic, grounded in the context of people's daily lives (Calnan, 1989, 1994; Calnan & Williams, 1991).

Medical sociology, subsequently, focused more on the meaning of a behaviour, the social contexts that inform the "style" of life a person chooses, and the effect of all of those on health-related practices (Calnan, 1994). Williams (1995), for instance, referenced the work of Pierre Bourdieu to explain the different dispositions and preferences that guide health-related practices between different social classes. Among the key insights was not so much that people from different social classes differ in their lifestyle choices—although they often do, as Calnan's (1990) study on food and consumption between middle-class and working-class women illustrated—but that irrespective of socio-economic circumstances health issues were typically engaged in unthinkingly, guided by implicit logic (Williams, 1995). It follows, so Williams (1995) argues, what Bourdieu (1977, 1990) called "*a feel for the game that works outside conscious control and discourse*," a predisposition that is derived from the fact that we do not think too hard about what we do because we do not have to.

We ought to pause here as our analysis of resistance to health messages has reached a point where explanations bifurcate into the topic of the next chapter, namely habitual behaviour. As we get closer to our definition for resistance, we shall see that despite close connections of resistance to ideas of agency and power, resistance is also robustly interlaced with social practice and practical consciousness.

Power and Agency

To understand the position of the concept of power, we need to go back to the above-mentioned shift in the new public health and health promotion discourse to impose individual responsibility on the preservation of good health and prevention of illness. What some socio-cultural studies on public health dealt with under the ideas of discipline or "bio-power" and health subjectivities (Briggs, 2003; Lupton, 1995) were notions of people being required "*to practice certain types of informed health behaviours and utilise health services appropriately, thereby implicitly reinforcing the expansion of health consumerism*" (Merrild et al., 2011).

Whereas we could ethically object to the idea of a consumerist production of health, the implicit requirement to live in a way that affords us to avoid the use of health services altogether does not conjure up ideas of resistance. Following good advice to go to one's doctor for preventative check-ups to not get so ill that one must see multiple medical experts later in a much worse state of health seems like a reasonable proposition.

Some studies (Dumas et al., 2014; Warin et al., 2015) argued that the lack of behaviour adoption has to do with a mismatch. Whereby the typical health promotion is oriented towards the prevention of future, intangible health complications, many people—especially disadvantaged groups—are faced with structural factors and short-term life and survival perspectives that render future-oriented campaigns irrelevant for lives shaped by immediacy (Merrild et al., 2011).

For instance, Satter (2007) demonstrated in her hierarchy of food needs model—a model derived from Abraham Maslow's theory of human motivation—how food consumption choice motivators follow certain needs states depending on life circumstances, whereby promoted nutritional healthy food choices are only chosen when "*one is in a position to achieve a desired physical, cognitive, or spiritual outcome.*" In simple terms, I choose healthy options if there is reliable access to affordable options.

Necessities and priority setting do explain to some extent why (some) people contest or ignore health recommendations. But if we recall Williams' (1995) notion of health-related behaviours as features of daily life routines, it implicitly suggests that people have developed and internalised certain routines. The answer to the origin of (routinised) actions may be found in Geertz' (1973) theory of the cultural process that emphasises the construction of meaning and subjectivities through symbolic processes embedded in the social world (Ortner, 2006). Understanding cultural formation as a relatively coherent body of symbols, meanings, and worldviews, it places social structures that operate on and shape the person to one side and a system of perceptions and practices that results from learning and experiences on the other. This dialectic between powerful social structures and human agency working back and forth in a dynamic relationship is the focus of practice theory, whose fundamental assumption is that culture (in a broad sense) constructs people as particular kinds of social actors but social actors—through their lived, variable practices—reproduce or transform the culture that made them. It is strongly associated with the French theorist and sociologist Pierre Bourdieu, whose ideas we have encountered above.

While agency is closely related to the concept of power—even if one only sees it as an idea of resistance to power—it is equally related to the concept of intentionality, where it describes people's purposes and desires towards what practice theorists call "culturally established projects" (Ortner, 2006). As Ortner (2006) continues:

> *The agency of projects is not necessarily about domination and resistance, although there may be some of that going on. It is about people having desires that grow out of their own structures of life, including very centrally their own structures of inequality; it is in short about people playing, or trying to play, their own serious games even as more powerful parties seek to devalue and even destroy them.* (p. 147)

What all of this translates to for health communication is that we ought to understand the lack of receptivity to a well-intended campaign not so much as a rebellious refusal to being told what to do and how to act, but rather an attempt to achieve or preserve one's own living conditions by converting official health information into actions conducive with one's own life to the degree it is possible. If we understand such health behaviour and subsequent actions as the result of one's own health narrative, then we can look at resistance as something Giroux (1992) termed an opposition or response to a "dominant" narrative. Hence, correctly interpreting the relationship between resistance and an alleged power of health promotion and prevention discourse opens a space where people's subjective experiences can be better understood (Hoffman, 1999).

Health Resistance Revisited

It may seem somewhat counterintuitive to venture an explanation for what appears to be a personal motivational act when we just argued that we ought not to regard it as a refusal to follow advice that improves health. However, it should become clearer now that health is a more complex topic to interact with than most promoters assume.

For one, personal health is not really a topic that most people think about, let alone talk about much unless they do not possess it any longer. As Williams (1995) explained, health is taken for granted and only discussed when someone is patently not healthy anymore. Accordingly, what we know as 'health-related-behaviour' (or the opposite thereof) are basically just features of daily routines that do not merit any conversation unless problems surface. Williams goes on to describe that when people are recruited for health communication research projects, what they end up talking about is what they think they should do rather than what they normally tend to do. It relates to what Giddens (1984) termed practical vs. discursive consciousness, with the two states having a complex interaction but being separate frames of mind. For now, we propose two preliminary clues: (1) Health is not a central topic in most (healthy) people's mind, and they only focus on it when either required or prompted. (2) Drawing conclusions from those prompted answers may result in a so-called boomerang effect, not so much because of contestations of the biomedical facts but rather because of the tone and positionality of the information/campaign and its sender.

In 2002, an article by Michele Crossley (2002a, b), a lecturer in behavioural science in the UK, appeared in the Health Education Journal, in which she reported on a phenomenon she called health resistance. It was aptly subtitled, the limits of contemporary health promotion. In it, she refers to her own and others' ethnographic research on various prevention behaviour interventions to explain how resistance to contemporary health promotion can be traced back to the linkage of physical well-being with cultural or moral right or wrong spurred by a desire for health and self-improvement.

This, of course, resembles Brehm's theory of psychological reactance (1981, 1966), i.e., an uneasy motivational state experienced by persons, who perceive a freedom to engage in a specific behaviour as threatened or in danger of being eliminated. He went on to argue that those people will often re-establish their freedoms by engaging in the opposite of the proscribed behaviour, known in social psychology as the 'boomerang effect.' Thus, if health messages are perceived as patronising, or worse, censorship, they may increase a motivation to engage in or continue with what health promoters have defined as the 'unhealthy' or 'risky' behaviour. Probably the use of the term 'risky' alone might make understandable why some people display a resistant behaviour since the definition of what constitutes high risk in a private behaviour was made by someone other than the targeted person.

Dowd et al. (1991) had shown that resistance can be understood as an individual personality trait, i.e., some people feel a higher need for freedom than others. However, Crossley (2001) also found cultural and social factors to play a role. The latter relates resistance to a group's values vis-à-vis institutions and organisational hierarchies, and subsequently scepticism towards ideas and messages emanating from such structures. Although those two concepts are naturally interlaced as individuals live in their respective cultural communities, it still makes sense to distinguish whether an act of resistance is a personal solitary one or a collective movement. For instance, someone being a closet smoker by herself is different from an entire neighbourhood refusing to vaccinate its children. While the former can hypothetically be explained and addressed with behavioural theories (which tend to focus on individual responses), the latter has elements of social movement theories and requires a different reply as they often are accompanied by suggestions for alternative courses of action to the prescribed one. We should add that no individual behaviour is entirely separated from its social environment.

Hence, it should be unsurprising that the last thoughts close a loop to previously mentioned arguments about meaning making of health and risk by individuals and social groups. In fact, Joffe (2002) challenged intrapersonal cognitive theories and models of risk perception and referred to social representation theory as a rubric to offer an alternative interpersonal understanding of people's responses to health promotion and health-related interventions. She argued that because "*the history and symbols held dear within particular social networks fashion [people's] representations of the health issues they face, [they] are difficult to change because they serve an identity protective function, rather than being products of faulty information processing*" (p. 153). So, instead of providing more information to rectify an assumed lack of knowledge, health promoters would be better off starting with mapping representational locations of audiences, which invariably includes interpersonal communication acts, or the "*permanent dialogue that people have with each other*" as Joffe called it. We will dive deeper into whether these explanations are connected to health communication in Chap. 7.

Communication Concerns

The importance of communication is best demonstrated by Crossley's findings that 'resistance' phenomena—as we mentioned above—mostly emerge in the context of a particular dialogical situation, where people are confronted with messages containing appeals and concrete instructions. As we discussed in the previous chapter, since communication does not fall into a social vacuum but is received and processed through individual and social prisms, health communicative barriers are typically based on ideological incompatibilities about personal health and the rhetorical significance of communication (Rimal & Lapinski, 2009). Fox's work (2002, 2006), for instance, showed how scientific language, most often used in health promotion, was interpreted by some members of the public as "how 'stupid and irrational' they are when they fail to engage in 'healthy' behaviours" (Fox, 2002).

These communicative barriers are specifically pronounced for disease prevention agendas, such as obesity, drinking/drink driving, or road safety. Here, they create an uneasy dialectic in communication, where positive health or well-being encouragements exist next to expert-driven warnings of future diseases or life risks, followed by subsequent instructions to prevent those. Besides the lack of congruence between those explanations and public responses (Putland et al., 2011), prevention communication sits in an uneasy place as far as reception is concerned. If it leans too far towards policy and regulation, it suffers from being considered paternalistic by creating an assumption that people cannot be trusted to make the healthy choice. If it aims to make communicative arguments for why and how individuals suffer from not yet having modified their behaviour, it often exposes itself to the equally unpleasant danger of being accused of condescension, including veiled accusations of victim blaming. Debates surrounding weight control campaigns that employed fat shaming (Lupton, 2015) or exacerbated fears of weight gain (Broom, 2008; Gjernes, 2010) illustrated this problem well. Before we move to discussing some new avenues, let's look at three examples:

D.A.R.E. Campaign (United States)

The U.S. American Drug Abuse Resistance Education, or D.A.R.E., was introduced into elementary school classrooms in 1983. They were based on police officers visiting middle schools and role-playing scenarios with the students, in which someone might offer them drugs or alcohol, and brainstorming ways to turn them down. Although this programme is no longer as widespread as it once was, it is still part of the curriculum in many school districts. The programme has proven ineffective. For instance, a study conducted at Indiana University of D.A.R.E.-exposed high school seniors with non-exposed seniors revealed no substantial differences in drug use between the two groups (Wysong & Wright, 1995). A ten-year follow-up study by the American Psychology Association equally found few differences between the two groups in terms of actual drug use, drug attitudes, or self-esteem, or differences in outcome success (Lynam et al., 1999).

Psychologist Dr. William Colson asserted in 1998 that D.A.R.E. increased drug awareness so that "*as they get a little older, they (students) become very curious about these drugs they've learned about from police officers*" (Laugesen, 1998). The evidence of a scientific research in 1998 indicated that by exposing young impressionable children to drugs, the programme, in fact, encouraged and nurtured drug use (Rosenbaum & Hanson, 1998). In the end, the programme failed by using the wrong communication approach. It has often been argued that the best approach to anti-drug campaigns towards teens is honesty and credibility. On the contrary, D.A.R.E. used exaggerations about the detrimental health effects of even less harmful drugs like marijuana. Teens dismissed these claims which, in turn, helped discredit the programme's overall efforts. In an age where drug use can be perceived as demonstrating independence and autonomy, language that simply discourages drug use as acts of weakness and stupidity are bound to encounter resistance. As a result of those studies, D.A.R.E. lost federal funding in 1998.

Headway's Cycle Helmet Campaign (UK)

In the mid-2010s, Headway, a brain injury not-for-profit, started a cycle safety campaign that essentially aimed at asking Britain's cyclist to wear bicycle helmets. Shortly, thereafter they also started lobbying for mandatory helmet laws. The campaign, "*Use your head - use a helmet*," was supported by "numerous peer-reviewed, published scientific studies and (…) well-respected professional bodies including the British Medical Association, the Association of Paediatric Emergency Medicine, the Bicycle Helmet Initiative Trust and numerous doctors and neurosurgeons across the UK" as well as the mention of a 2016 UK study of over 60,000 cyclists which found "compelling evidence that wearing a cycle helmet reduces risk of serious head injury by almost 70% and fatal head injury by 65%" ("Cycle Safety," 2017).

Although helmet laws exist in other countries (e.g., Australia has a helmet law since the 1990s) and so may seem for those citizens to be a no-brainer, the campaign experienced backlash from various groups, many of those cycling clubs and associations. Among the counterarguments are discouragement from cycling altogether (Dole, 2018), a missed approach to working on a better cycling or road infrastructure, and a wrong sense of safety (Walker, 2017).

Besides seemingly valid arguments such as true cycling safety not coming from a helmet but creating a road system (such as in the Netherlands and Scandinavia) that insulates vulnerable cyclists more from fast-moving road traffic, Nick Hussey, the founder of a British cycle clothing company, Vulpine was quoted in Walker's article as saying that the helmet debate reminds him of paternalistic overreach: "[It's like I march] *into a bar and snatch a third or fourth pint of beer from a random drinker's lips, yelling, 'Stop drinking or you will die!' That's more or less what the infamous helmet debate has become. Shouty strangers shouting at other shouty strangers for choices that don't affect the first shouty stranger's life. It's a bit weird*" (Hussey, as quoted in Walker, 2017).

While even the British Medical Association advocates the compulsory use of helmets, there are no cycling helmet laws in the UK today and any suggestions for change are fought by Cycling UK, among other groups. This example is reminiscent of the trials and tribulations of another safety device effort, namely automobile seatbelts. In their *Global Status Report on Road Safety* (2009), the WHO found that despite the proven risk reductions "nearly one of every four countries, for which data are available, have a seatbelt wearing rate of less than 50%." Fifty years after the first automobiles fitted with three-point seatbelts left the factory floors, there is still widespread resistance to using them despite numerous public awareness campaigns.

A Decade of Obesity Campaigns (Australia 2011–2018)

In late 2010, the Sydney Morning Herald newspaper quoted a report from the Productivity Commission, which found "*evidence that many schemes to prevent childhood obesity have failed to make a significant dent in the girths of young Australians*" (Metherell, 2010). The 170-page report had looked at 27 different programmes and campaigns, aimed to curb childhood obesity, and concluded that the causes of obesity are so complex that no effective intervention has been found yet. It followed this up with a call to restrict junk food marketing and improve package labelling. Two years later, a similar article (Stark, 2012) called Australia's obesity strategy a "wasteful failure."

Given that the so-called obesity epidemic occurs across population segments—and hence different cultures and values—it is not easy to ascertain the exact reasons for campaign failures towards any one group, aside from over-employing rather passive unidirectional media campaign approaches. In 2011, the U.S. American team of Walls and colleagues did provide a reasonable explanation that most likely applies to all groups, stating that: (a) campaigns are too individualised, (b) campaigns suffer from an uneasy confluence of health benefits with the social desirability of thinness, and (c) campaigns have an over-emphasis on educational efforts, contributing to inequalities in obesity reduction. They championed community-based efforts which "provide incentives for healthy eating and increased physical activity" (Walls et al., 2011), something Australia-based research teams reiterated (e.g., Nicholls et al., 2014).

In Australia, a 2011 review of mediated campaigns oriented towards obesity prevention found unsurprisingly that, on average, about two-thirds of target groups recall the main message but fewer change their attitudes or knowledge, and fewer still change their behaviour (reported in: Jones, 2018). Alas, it did not stop a diversity of relatively short-term, unbranded, and inconsistent campaigns, such as 'Unplug and Play' (2011), 'Swap it, don't stop it' (2012), 'Live lighter' (2014), or 'Move it Australia' (2018), to be launched in succession.

Granted, there have been attempts to get to the origins of this inertia. Obesity prevention research (Baum & Fisher, 2014; Nichols et al., 2013) pointed to disconnects in delivery, i.e., what channels campaign creators choose (or not choose, when we consider the relative higher effectiveness of community-based efforts) to reach target groups, and message content, i.e., what campaign creators think people want to hear and what people respond to. As we will explore in more detail in later chapters, a particular formula dominates obesity prevention planning, which goes like this: individuals are responsible for their own weight health status, but they lack the required information about health risks. Only by providing this information widely (usually via some form of media) will behaviour change occur. Hence, information must be communicated in a way that triggers change reactions (Lupton, 2014). As I have argued before, what this fails to take into consideration is peoples' real-life socio-economic and cultural environments, let alone the personal values people compare with what they encounter in obesity messages.

While admittedly each health issue and each individual campaign copes with its own detailed barriers and issues, what I hope these examples have brought into sharper focus is a general problem in communicating health and disease prevention. Whereas health communication happens in varying degrees of formal, semi-formal, and informal contexts, most health communication campaign practice focuses on formal settings and linear communication flows, such as mass media campaigns or, to a lesser extent, medical staff-to-patient communication (Silk et al., 2011). Focusing on so-called instrumental messages and goals, health communicators often neglect the identity and relational goals of everyday communication and behaviours (Welch Cline, 2011).

In other words, often disregarded social realities and norms have a stronger influence on communication and response than the more readily used variables of health knowledge or traditionally defined individual beliefs. As the third example has shown, disparities between expert knowledge on obesity and public practices in relation to the health risks posed by obesity reflects an unrealistic expectation placed in the predominant models of obesity communication (such as the individual attitude modification approach) that seem difficult to translate into practice (Medvedyuk et al., 2018). Yet, these models still dominate in agencies charged with the communication of expert knowledge, organisations that span numerous substantive domains such as science communication, risk, as well as many health concerns. They generally assume that once people have assimilated expert knowledge and are sufficiently motivated to follow the calls-to-action, they will attempt to adopt the recommended behaviour accordingly. However, it has been robustly argued that such models suffer from ignoring relevant elements, such as the role of trust/ sympathy towards experts and their knowledge as well as thoughts about a health entity's intention, the social processes entailed in assimilating said expert knowledge, or the complex relation between lifestyle and embedded health practices, largely shaped by one's habitus and socialisation (Halkier, 2015; Shove et al., 2012), let alone life circumstances.

Interpretation of Meaning in Health Communication

A body of studies on health promotion (Haines et al., 2004; Rychetnik & Wise, 2004; Rychetnik et al., 2002) has pointed out that a different understanding of the causes of disease and maintenance of good health within the population could reduce the tension between current theory-based intervention approaches and existing social and cultural complexities and structural difficulties, especially for disadvantaged groups.

As argued in the first chapter, health communication can offer insights into the significance of language choice, meaning, and understanding and provide a differently natured interpretation of 'transaction' as is common with the medical knowledge transfer approach. With social contexts providing certain norms and labels for communicating a particular health issue, language provides both a frame for this issue as well as networks of meaning. A more socio-cultural perspective of the representation of health and healthcare (Hall, 2005) will reveal communication's capability as a signal carrier for personal values and mission. If resistance can be understood as a breakdown in the dialogical process, subsequently leading to a lack of motivation to comply with the appeal, then improving the dialogical process should logically help to improve issues of resistance.

To that end, different models, such as social representation and practice models, which can identify the tensions between health campaign messages and everyday social practices (see e.g., Holland et al., 2015) show great potential to directly address current barriers to better intergroup communication. Pointing to the idea that virtually all human knowledge is based on stories constructed around past experiences, and that new experiences are interpreted in terms of old stories (Howarth, 2011), they can form a foundation for creating a system of common understanding, concepts, and ideas that have special meaning for a group, known as a communicative frame.

To an extent, I can understand that the average professional in public health promotion may look at what I am about to describe as some esoteric blather that has little connection to the time- and task-restricted efforts to facilitate lifestyle improvements. But note that we are not only already relying on socio-psychological interpretation of human thought and behaviour when constructing campaigns but that all human communication is creating and the result of social and self-representation. In addition, unlike what cognitivist models presuppose, people do not function as information processors who spent mental energy in solving causal theorems (Abelson, 1976; Newell & Simon, 1972). Instead, people mostly engage what Bruner (1986) termed narrative thinking. That is, they look for coherence in a message or story. He used the short sentence "the king died and then the queen died" to explain that when people encounter this statement, they look for likely connections between the two events, speculating on agents, intentions, situations, instruments while simultaneously experiencing some reaction towards the story such as grief, suspicion of foul play, etc. (c.f. László, 1997). Narrative thinking requires stories that construct two psychological domains, or as Bruner (1986) calls them landscapes, namely elements of action (agents, intentions/goals, situation, instrument) and elements of consciousness (plotting what the story actors know, think, or feel, as well as what they do not know, think, or feel). These then provide anchors for our self- and group-identities, as well as our self-representation, help us make sense of our world, and give us models for our thoughts and behaviours.

This human capacity to engage with and live a story is amply used by literature, film and, in a certain sub-genre, the news media (Iyengar, 1987; Oatley, 1992). Yet, health messages often fail to see the power of the narrative in everyday real life of social groups, where group identity is formed and re-formed through joint activities, which in turn reemphasise the experience of togetherness. Only occasionally do we encounter mediated campaigns where an unhealthy behaviour is displayed as part of a communal life story (e.g., the Australian National Tobacco Campaign (2017), targeting its Aboriginal population, titled "Don't make smokes your story") or where a generational story is told to explain an unhealthy behaviour to offer a solution (e.g., the Australian Drinkwise (2008) campaign, titled "Kids absorb your drinking").

The relevance of a narrative lies in its relatability by the receiver. Far more important than historical or scientific accuracy is the evoking of a lived experience that includes convincing explanations and resolutions to life's mysteries and struggles (Spence, 1982). In fact, this approach is the one used by psychotherapy to restore the mental health of a patient.

This, in the end, gets us to a probable explanation of why health messages are resisted or rejected, and a possible answer to that dilemma. Most appeals in health communication are created in a cause-and-effect relationship, and any story plot that may surround it serves to emphasise or embellish this logical sequence. Often, logical arguments and/or evidence further assists in this logical arc. Yet, if we study narratives more closely—as we will do later—we find that narrative causality does not operate in this kind of relationship but that acts (or, as we may call it here, behaviours) result from personal intentions or desires. These intentions, however, do not cause the action/behaviour but merely provide reasons or motives for it (László, 2008).

What follows from that is that human narratives (the stories people tell each other) are ambiguous as there is no one logical truth. Instead, the goal is consistency of the story and its meaning with life experiences or group/community dynamics. In simple terms, the story fits with how I or we understand myself/ourselves and the world around me/us.

So, in lieu of focusing on objective knowledge and independence from its subjective interpretations, a hermeneutic approach, which does precisely that—namely emphasising subjective interpretations of meanings of texts, art, culture, social phenomena, and thinking—could be a way forward in having a real dialogue with health communication receivers. When we talk in this context about the interpreter's understanding of the text, we do not talk about literacy skills but merely the personal decoding of this text.

In other words, our discipline has so far mainly focused on figuring out whether a message recipient has properly decoded the sender's intentions. This does include both the previous ideas of literacy/cognitive ability as well as a person's cognitive functioning/pathway. In short, we aim to see how we can bring the reading of the text in line with the intention for having it sent so the desired reaction can or will occur. Instead, we may ought to establish real relationships between reader, text, and context. Since no interpretation or description is entirely independent from the effects of the receiver's experiences, pre-suppositions, and projections of his or her personal values and expectations, getting to the core of not only how a text (or shall I say, story) is read but also what conclusions are drawn from it and why should not only reduce resistance barriers but also afford us to understand why those exist in the first place. In the end, any communication resulting from it can arrive at the word's etymological origin, namely a way to *share meaning*, which is the foundation of communicative relationships.

References

Abelson, R. (1976). Scripts in attitude formation and decision making. In J. Carrol & J. Payne (Eds.), *Cognition and social behavior* (pp. 33–45). Erlbaum.

Bacchi, C. (1999). *Women, policy and politics: The construction of policy problems*. Sage.

Baum, F., & Fisher, M. (2014). Why behavioural health promotion endures despite its failure to reduce health inequities. *Sociology of Health & Illness, 36*(2), 213–225.

Bourdieu, P. (1977). *Outline of a theory of practice*. Cambridge University Press.

Bourdieu, P. (1990). *The logic of practice*. Polity Press.

Brehm, J. (1966). *A theory of psychological reactance.* Academic Press.
Brehm, J., & Brehm, S. (1981). *Psychological reactance.* Wiley.
Briggs, C. (2003). Why nation-states and journalists can't teach people to be healthy: Power and pragmatic miscalculation in public discourses on health. *Medical Anthropology Quarterly, 17*(2), 287–321.
Broom, D. (2008). Hazardous good intentions? Unintended consequences of the project of prevention. *Health Sociology Review, 17*(2), 129–140.
Bruner, J. (1986). *Actual minds, possible worlds.* Harvard University Press.
Calnan, M. (1989). Control over health and patterns of health-related behavior. *Social Science and Medicine, 24,* 435–455.
Calnan, M. (1994). 'Lifestyle' and its social significance. In G. L. Albrecht (Ed.), *Advances in medical sociology* (Vol. 4). JAI Press Inc.
Calnan, M., & Williams, S. (1991). Style of life and the salience of health: An exploratory study of health-related practices in households from differing socio-economic circumstances. *Sociology of Health & Illness, 13,* 506–529.
Crossley, M. (2001). "Resistance" and health promotion. *Health Education Journal, 60*(3), 197–204.
Crossley, M. (2002a). Resistance to health promotion: A preliminary comparative investigation of British and Australian students. *Health Education, 102*(6), 289–299.
Crossley, M. (2002b). Introduction to the symposium 'health resistance': The limits of contemporary health promotion. *Health Education Journal, 61*(2), 101–112.
Cycle Safety-Headway's 'Use your head-use a helmet' Campaign. (2017). https://www.headway.org.uk/get-involved/campaigns/cycle-safety/
Dole, N. (2018, January 26). *UK cyclists fight campaign to make helmets compulsory.* https://www.abc.net.au/news/2018-01-26/uk-cyclists-fight-compulsory-helmet-campaign/9345708
Dowd, E., Milne, C., & Wise, S. (1991). The therapeutic reactance scale: A measure of psychological reactance. *Journal of Counselling & Development, 69,* 541–545.
Drinkwise. (2008). *Kids absorb your drinking.* https://drinkwise.org.au/our-work/parents-campaign/#
Dumas, A., Robitaille, J., & Jette, S. (2014). Lifestyle as a choice of necessity: Young women, health and obesity. *Social Theory & Health, 12,* 138–158.
Eagle, L., Bulmer, S., & Hawkins, J. (2003). *The obesity epidemic: Complex causes, controversial cures. Technical Report.* Massey University Press.

Fox, N. (2002). What a 'risky' body can do: Why people's health choices are not all based in evidence. *Health Education Journal, 61*, 166–179.
Fox, N., & Ward, K. (2006). Health identities: From expert patient to resisting. *Health, 10*(4), 461–479.
Geertz, C. (1973). *The interpretation of cultures*. Basic Books.
Giroux, H. (1992). *Border crossings: Cultural workers and the politics of education*. Routledge.
Gjernes, T. (2010). Facing resistance to health advice. *Health, Risk & Society, 12*(5), 471–489.
Haines, A., Kuruvilla, S., & Borchert, M. (2004). Bridging the implementation gap be-tween knowledge and action for health. *Bulletin of the World Health Organisation, 82*, 724–732.
Halkier, B. (2015). Mundane science use in a practice theoretical perspective: Different understandings of the relations between citizen-consumers and public communication initiatives build on scientific claims. *Public Understanding of Science, 26*(1), 40–54.
Hall, P. (2005). Interprofessional teamwork: Professional cultures as barriers. *Journal of Interprofessional Care, 19*(Suppl 1), 188–196.
Hoffman, D. (1999). Turning power inside out: Reflections on resistance from the (anthropological) field. *International Journal of Qualitative Studies in Education, 12*(6), 671–687.
Holland, K., Blood, R., Thomas, S., & Lewis, S. (2015). Challenging stereotypes and legitimating fat: An analysis of obese people's views on news media reporting guidelines and promoting body diversity. *Journal of Sociology, 51*(2), 431–445.
Howarth, C. (2011). Representations, identity and resistance in communication. In D. Hook, B. Franks, & M. Bauer (Eds.), *The social psychology of communication* (pp. 153–168). Palgrave Macmillan.
Iyengar, S. (1987). Television news and citizens' explanations of national affairs. *The American Political Science Review, 81*, 815–832.
Joffe, H. (2002). Representations of health risks: What social psychology can offer health promotion. *Health Education Journal, 61*(2), 153–165.
Jones, S. (2018, August). Will the government's new 'move it' exercise campaign move us or lose us? *The Conversation*. https://theconversation.com/will-the-governments-new-move-it-exercise-campaign-move-us-or-lose-us-100969
László, J. (1997). Narrative organisation of social representations. *Papers on Social Representations, 6*(2), 155–172.
László, J. (2008). *The science of stories: An introduction to narrative psychology*. Routledge.

Laugesen, W. (1998). *Dec 4*. The dire consequences of D.A.R.E.
Lupton, D. (1995). *The imperative of health: Public health and the regulated body*. Sage.
Lupton, D. (2014). "How do you measure up?" assumptions about "obesity" and health-related behaviors and beliefs in two Australian "obesity" prevention campaigns. *Fat Studies, 3*(1), 32–44.
Lupton, D. (2015). The pedagogy of disgust: The ethical, moral and political implications of using disgust in public health campaigns. *Critical Public Health, 25*(1), 4–14.
Lynam, D., Milich, R., Zimmerman, R., Novak, S., Logan, T., Martin, C., Leukefeld, C., & Clayton, R. (1999). Project DARE: No effects at 10-year follow-up. *Journal of Consulting and Clinical Psychology, 67*(4), 590–593.
Medvedyuk, S., Ali, A., & Raphael, D. (2018). Ideology, obesity and the social determinants of health: A critical analysis of the obesity and health relation ship. *Critical Public Health, 28*(5), 573–585.
Merrild, C., Andersen, R., Risør, M., & Vedsted, P. (2011). Resisting "reason": A comparative anthropological study of social differences and resistance toward health promotion and illness prevention in Denmark. *Medical Anthropology Quarterly, 31*(2), 218–236.
Metherell, M. (2010, October 26). *Heavyweight campaigns failing children*. https://www.smh.com.au/lifestyle/health-and-wellness/heavyweight-campaigns-failing-children-20101025-170ws.html
Miles, A., Rapoport, L., Wardle, J., Afuape, T., & Duman, M. (2001). Using the mass-media to target obesity: An analysis of the characteristics and reported behaviour change of participants in the BBC's 'Fighting Fat, Fighting Fit' campaign. *Health Education Research, 16*(3), 357–372.
National Tobacco Campaign. (2017). *Don't make smokes your story*. Australian Government Department of Health. https://www.quitnow.gov.au/internet/quitnow/publishing.nsf/Content/stakeholder-toolkit
Newell, A., & Simon, H. (1972). *Human problem solving*. Prentice-Hall.
Nichols, M., Reynolds, R., Waters, E., Gill, T., King, L., Swinburn, B., & Allender, S. (2013). Community-based efforts to prevent obesity: Australia-wide survey of projects. *Health Promotion Journal of Australia, 24*(2), 111–117.
Nicholls, L., Lewis, A., Petersen, S., Swinburn, B., Moodie, M., & Millar, L. (2014). Parental encouragement of healthy behaviors: Adolescent weight status and health-related quality of life. *BMC Public Health, 14*, 369. https://doi.org/10.1186/1471-2458-14-369.
Oatley, K. (1992). *Best laid schemes*. Cambridge University Press.

Ortner, S. (2006). *Anthropology and social theory: Culture, power, and the acting subject*. Duke University Press.
Putland, C., Baum, F., & Ziersch, A. (2011). From causes to solutions - insights from lay knowledge about health inequalities. *BMC Public Health, 1*, 67.
Rimal, R., & Lapinski, M. (2009). Why health communication is important in public health. *Bulletin of the World Health Organization, 87*, 247–247.
Rosenbaum, D., & Hanson, G. (1998). Assessing the effects of school-based drug education: A six-year multilevel analysis of project D.A.R.E. *Journal of Research in Crime and Delinquency, 35*(4), 381–412.
Rychetnik, L., Frommer, M., Hawe, P., & Shiell, A. (2002). Criteria for evaluating evidence on public health interventions. *Journal of Epidemiology & Community Health, 56*, 119–127.
Rychetnik, L., & Wise, M. (2004). Advocating evidence-based health promotion: Reflections and a way forward. *Health Promotion International, 19*(2), 247–257.
Satter, E. (2007). Hierarchy of food needs. *Journal of Nutrition Education and Behavior, 39*(5), S187–S188.
Shilling, C. (2002). Culture, the "sick role" and the consumption of health. *British Journal of Sociology, 53*(4), 621–638.
Shove, E., Pantzar, M., & Watson, M. (2012). *The dynamics of social practice*. Sage.
Silk, K., Atkin, C., & Salmon, C. (2011). Developing effective media campaigns for health promotion. In T. Thompson, R. Parrott, & J. Nussbaum (Eds.), *The Routledge handbook of health communication* (2nd ed., pp. 230–246). Routledge.
Spence, D. (1982). *Narrative truth and historical truth*. W.W. Norton and Company.
Stark, J. (2012, December 2). *Obesity strategy a 'wasteful failure'*. https://www.smh.com.au/national/obesity-strategy-a-wasteful-failure-20121201-2ao3x.html
Walker, P. (2017, March 22). *The big bike helmet debate: You don't make it safe by forcing cyclists to dress for urban warfare*. https://www.theguardian.com/lifeandstyle/2017/mar/21/bike-helmet-cyclists-safe-urban-warfare-wheels
Walls, H., Peeters, A., Proietto, J., & McNeil, J. (2011). Public health campaigns and obesity – A critique. *BMC Public Health, 11*, 136–143.
Wardle, J., Rapoport, L., Miles, A., Afuape, T., & Duman, M. (2001). Mass education for obesity prevention: The penetration of the BBC's 'Fighting Fat, Fighting Fit' campaign. *Health Education Research, 16*(3), 343–355.

Warin, M., Zivkovic, T., Moore, V., Ward, P., & Jones, M. (2015). Short horizons and obesity futures: Disjunctures between public health interventions and everyday temporalities. *Social Science & Medicine, 128*, 309–315.
Welch Cline, R. (2011). Everyday interpersonal communication and health. In T. Thompson, R. Parrott, & J. Nussbaum (Eds.), *The Routledge handbook of health communication* (2nd ed., pp. 285–313). Routledge.
Whitehead, D., & Russell, G. (2004). How effective are health education programmes – Resistance, reactance, rationality and risk? *International Journal of Nursing Studies, 41*, 163–172.
WHO. (2009). *Global status report on road safety: Time for action*. World Health Organization.
Williams, S. (1995). Theorizing class, health and lifestyle: Can Bourdieu help us? *Sociology of Health and Illness, 17*(5), 577–604.
Wysong, E., & Wright, D. (1995). A decade of DARE: Efficacy, politics and drug education. *Sociological Focus, 28*(3), 283–311.

3

Creatures of Habit: Automatic Health Behaviour

Overview

When we talk in health promotion about the behavioural decisions people make to follow or resist advice or interventions, we tend to imply a thoughtful choice. The implicit assumption behind a health message recipient's compliant or resistant response is that of a cognitive act about the upcoming response and any consequences that may ensue from it. It is the standard logic flow behind most official health communication campaigns, especially if any cognition-based model is the theoretic foundation for the strategies and tactics in the campaign effort.

Yet, often, we do not really think our actions through all that much, if at all. We often either execute ingrained habitual patterns because we 'always did this,' act in the so-called 'spur of the moment' or did so because it felt right. In either case, if we were ever queried about the precise motivator for the behavioural choice after we displayed it, we had a hard time explaining in enough detail why we acted that way or chose this option. Consider these few examples:

O. Werder, *Transformational Health Communication*,
https://doi.org/10.1007/978-981-99-9606-3_3

1. People, who usually don't drink excessively when alone, feel compelled to imbibe when surrounded by drinkers, who encourage to join them to 'have fun together.'
2. In my neighbourhood, I often see on Saturday mornings groups of quite serious cyclists (judging from their semi-professional outfit and equipment) concluding their weekly bike ride at the village cafè for some lattès and pastries to chat the rest of the Saturday morning away before going home. Apparently, the preceding exercise evens out the increased calorie intake.
3. Reflect on the scores of people who mindlessly grab a cigarette, an alcoholic drink, an ice cream, or anything that makes them feel good or better in order to either celebrate a personal victory or extirpate their sorrows, frustration, fear, or anger.
4. Finally, a lot of people questioned by police over their violation of enforced COVID-19 restrictions were not actually purposeful virus deniers but momentarily chose to do (e.g., gather in larger groups) or not do (e.g., wearing a face mask) something out of habit or emotionally.

This list could go on but what these examples have in common is that a behaviour has occurred without much reason or consideration, let alone purposeful denial or rejection of the cause of the opposing counsel. For these types of behavioural patterns an attempt to influence the individual's cognitive decision ability and leaning is ill-fated to work. There is a likelihood that, if interviewed about healthy behaviour, most of the people in our examples would agree with encountered arguments about making good choices and may already make those in other aspects of their daily routines or lives.

Accordingly, in this chapter we try to untangle the complex world of habits, intuition, ad-hoc choices, and affective reactions, and how to best include them in health communication.

Habits

When we are very young, most of us are told by our parents that we should develop good habits. But what is a habit? Over a century ago, the *American Journal of Psychology* defined it as a "*more or less fixed way of thinking, willing, or feeling acquired through previous repetition of a mental experience*" (Andrews, 1903). That is, it encompasses all behaviours that we do not (have to) think about much and/or do subconsciously because we have repeated them so often and regularly that they have become routine. But that is not all. In the late nineteenth century, the psychologist and philosopher William Hall stated, "*all our life, so far as it has definite form, is but a mass of habits*" (1899). In other words, much of our daily behaviours or choices are not repetitive deliberate actions but habitual and this includes all sorts of behaviours, not just those we would like to internalise.

If we think about our myriads of daily actions from the moment we get out of bed to the moment we fall asleep, all of us follow particular patterns regarding personal hygiene, dressing, taking meals, travelling to and from work, organising our chores, hobbies, choice of TV programmes, and the order and combination of all of these that we find hard to explain and describe when directly asked.

In our health communication course, we invite students to think about and discuss their unplanned actions—roughly around the time when we start to discuss the standard health behaviour theories. It is fascinating—but not too surprising—to see how students grapple with an answer or even make sense of this idea. Like everyone else, they do not give much thought to these small supposedly meaningless acts. And while it is probably accurate to say that a single habit, such as tying your left shoe before your right shoe, does not carry much weight, in their totality and chronology of occurrence in relation to all aspects of our lives they have a huge impact on it, including on our health. As Duhigg (2012) in his intriguing work on habits noted, a 2006 study by Duke University found that over 40% of people's daily actions were not the result of decision but habits, many of which with potentially direct implications for personal health and hygiene.

The Bias of Intuition

The million-dollar question of any prevention communication is, of course, how to engage people, who at the time of message encounter do not suffer (yet) from any specific disease or ailment. Given that the intended targets of preventative communication have no current ill-health condition, pondering their health ranks relatively low on their everyday agenda, and in the wake, messages that warn of possible future negative effects are not often retained in memory, at least not to the extent that a content expert wishes or assumes.

Aggravating this predisposition of indifference is a process we all engage in daily for most things we encounter. Most of our daily actions—or our life's journey and social behaviours as a whole—is directed by our impulsive, automated system, or, to use Kahneman's (2012) terminology, our System 1. Unlike our reflective system that follows a stepwise flow of logical reasoning to assess an idea or stimulus, our impulsive system that, by the way, controls our actions far more often, operates through activating habits, known as schemata, that require little cognitive effort.

The idea of schemas goes back to gestalt psychology, specifically to Jean Piaget's (1936) theory of cognitive development. He argued that our schemas form basic building blocks of knowledge and behaviours from our past experiences or, to borrow from Wadsworth (2004), mental "index cards" that help us to react swiftly to incoming stimuli or information. For example, most of us developed a particular schema of seeing our regular physician from early childhood, which we retain as standard behavioural practice. It typically includes making an appointment with the reception desk, checking in on the day and then waiting in the waiting area, later, when called in, sitting in the visitor's chair and explaining our health concern and symptoms, following the doctor's orders during the individual checks, listening to her diagnosis and conclusions, filling the medical script if given one, paying (if required) and leaving, followed by complying with any other follow-up request like seeing a specialist, taking a blood test, etc. So, whenever we have a similar medical appointment situation in future times, we retrieve this schema from memory and apply it to the subsequent visit. In addition, the communicative relationship that we experience during those formative stages (discussion among equals, silent listening) also transfers to future encounters.

What is interesting and relevant about all that is the heuristic fashion, by which schematic worldviews get applied. If new information or impressions fall within an individual's schema, they will easily be added to it. If they do not, the new information either tends to get ignored or re-interpreted to minimise the effect on one's schema. Both tendencies lead to what is known as confirmation and disconfirmation bias (O'Sullivan & Durso, 1984; Stanovich et al., 2013), i.e., the recall and interpretation of information that confirms pre-existing beliefs as well as the creation of higher standards for evidence that contradicts those. Among other reasons, it helps explain discordant behaviour during the early stages of the COVID-19 epidemic with some reacting to it like they would to relatable virus infections, like the annual flu.

This mental process has also direct implications for the adoption of digital technology in healthcare and prevention. For instance, in 2018 a new healthcare IT company, called Med Advisor, started its operation in Australia, providing a fully digital end-to-end experience for handling medical scripts for prescribed medication (people can download their service to their mobile devices via an app). In principle, improving the interaction between pharmacies, patients, drug manufacturers, doctors, and governments is beneficial and speeds things up. However, adoption has been slow as the whole process is a new way (or schema) in getting and taking medication. It appears that many people find it strange to outsource this known process to a digital service (we can see a similar scenario in digital banking neatly dividing enthusiastic younger tech generations from hesitant less tech-enthusiastic older ones). I have also heard recently from my local pharmacist that this lack of uptake has them also move away from promoting and endorsing it.

This is not to say that schemata are entirely rigid. Piaget deftly explained in his discussion of cognitive assimilation vs. accommodation how new shortcuts (schemata) get created in the case of new information not fitting in any current schema. So, there is some movement in our intuitive brain and decision-making efforts. However, using our mental heuristics to engage memories for assessing new stimuli impedes the acceptance of new information, especially when it contradicts current beliefs, including held stereotypes. It can also lead to memory distortion, where information or events are recalled that did not happen or did not happen in a particular way, simply because the memorised version is more in line with a held schema (Tuckey & Brewer, 2003). For example, there are studies (e.g., Higgs & Thomas, 2016) that have discussed the social influence of dining in company, where deviations from habitual eating patterns (kinds or amounts of food) are explained away or simply ignored considering the social dynamics. In one of our ongoing studies on people's travel health habits we observed that people had a skewed self-assessment when it comes to their planning and preparedness for health and emergency situations. A similar example is the debate surrounding face masks to protect against virus transmission. In countries, such as Japan or China, where the practice of wearing a mask to prevent the spread of an infectious disease has become a common habit, we do not see the kind of contortions and debates by government officials and members of the public as we have experienced in many Western countries, when this did become a strong suggestion or enforceable act in the COVID-19 pandemic.

Over the past decades, the process of biased unintentional information processing has been studied by a range of disciplines from environmental psychology to behavioural economics. It included in-depth research on a host of cognitive biases such as:

1. Wishful thinking, i.e., the overestimation of the likelihood of desirable events (e.g., Aue et al., 2012)
2. The Pollyanna principle, i.e., the selective favouring to process pleasant over unpleasant information (e.g., Jones, 2014)
3. The overconfidence effect, i.e., the overestimation of one's knowledge and ability to predict realistic future outcomes (e.g., Hoffrage, 2004)
4. The confirmation bias, i.e., the favouring of information that confirms previously held beliefs or hypotheses (e.g., Nickerson, 1998)
5. Positive test strategies, i.e., a type of cost-benefit analysis whose main objective is to avoid the costliest error (e.g., Zuckerman et al., 1995) and
6. Biased risk assessment, best exemplified by the well-known prospect theory (Kahneman & Tversky, 1979), i.e., the personal weighing of gains and losses, e.g., of a preventative test, based on message frames and expected utility or benefit (Schwartz et al., 2008).

All these tendencies to subjectively collect, interpret, and retain (health) information affect a person's information processing in a way that results in a behavioural response that cannot easily be predicted by rational processing models.

Further, a related effect whereby someone's distorted self-diagnosis of a condition or state alters that person's behaviour in a way that the expected result really happens is known as the Placebo effect. It goes back to the self-fulfilling prophecy, discussed by Merton (1948). Studies have shown that people's self-rating about their health has affected their physical health and mortality more than standard biomedical indicators, such as blood pressure, BMI, activity levels, or cholesterol (Idler & Kasl, 1995; Mossey & Shapiro, 1982). In another study by the Norwegian University of Science and Technology the research team found that teenage girls who were not fat, but felt they were, were more likely to become overweight as adults (Cuypers et al., 2012).

This instinctive adjustment of one's behaviour to one's own expectations is further compounded by the phenomenon of adjusting one's responses and self-beliefs according to what one thinks others think about them. Whereas this does not typically end up in *allodoxaphobia*, i.e., the anxiety of hearing other people's opinion about oneself, regular exposure to stigmatising messages has been shown to threaten the social identity of individuals who may already have negative self-perceptions regarding a particular condition, such as, for instance, weight management (see e.g., Major et al., 2014). Those critical voices for many come from mediated environments, which because of the explosive growth of the digital media have not only proliferated in recent years but at the same time have given room to voices that were often in direct opposition to each other, such as is the case in the body weight/obesity debate (e.g., Lupton, 2017).

It should be clear by now that communication plays a critical role in the creation or proliferation of these effects but can likewise be a valid contributor of correcting them.

Communication Fallacies

As we alluded to earlier, in public health promotion the explanation for the causes of human behaviour is based on the widespread assumption that they result from an assessment of the value and utility of an action. Hence, the standard choice for message content includes credible, science-backed facts, transposed into logical cause-effect sequences for right and wrong action. This message frame is, of course, a derivative of the earlier assumption. If people logically assess their actions, then they equally logically process messages.

This may explain why many health marketing efforts make use of the (cognitive) behaviourist theories, we mentioned earlier (such as the Health Belief Model or Theory of Planned Behaviour), as those emphasise a logical cognitive path towards the ultimate behavioural response. If the desired behaviour does not occur—or is different from modelled expectations—one typical explanation is that message recipients lack the necessary knowledge or education to engage in the act. It has sped up the growth of whole subfields within public health, known as health literacy and health education. I should add that lack of understanding, whether the result of personal education levels by recipients or chosen complexity in the delivery of an appeal, is at times indeed the reason behind lack of compliance. I have more to say about that later.

An alternate foundational approach to explaining the effect of health interventions goes back to early twentieth-century psychoanalysis (especially Freudian ideas), i.e., the existence of multiple determining processes, some being rational, others consisting of basic drives and unconscious acting. Following this conceptual idea, this stream of psychology has contributed multiple explanations for systematic/reasoning vs. peripheral/heuristics processing (Chaiken & Trope, 1999; Epstein, 1991; Fazio, 1990; Petty & Cacioppo, 1986; Smith & DeCoster, 2000) in the past three decades. However, the processes described in these models focus mostly on judgements and information processing instead of behavioural consequences and, hence, do not provide a massive melioration compared with rational models of human behaviour (Strack & Deutsch, 2004).

What both approaches share—and what subsequently informs health message content and form—is the assumption that human behaviour follows predictable patterns akin to other organic patterns and hence can be reduced to its elements and quantified. The predictability of behaviour is determined, at least in part, by previous behavioural responses. It seems more apropos, though, to allow for a combination of feeling and thinking, based on individual perceptions and beliefs about events, life conditions, and such amorphous states such as love, fulfilment, self-worth, and autonomy that differ across time and persons.

It is the focus of a movement in psychology, known as humanistic psychology, which started in the United States in the early 1960s (Moss,

2014). It is intricately connected to the works of one scholar, Abraham Maslow, whose theory of self-actualisation served as the foundation for the growth of the sub-discipline. While it has spawned new approaches to therapy (e.g., gestalt and constructivist therapy), its influence on a wider application by other disciplines has remained comparatively sporadic. Maslow's original work of the hierarchy of needs, which he introduced in his paper "A theory of human motivation" (Maslow, 1943), is probably one of the better-known and easier-to-understand theories of human motivation. It has been my experience that many students are aware of its basic premises. However, routine application of the major ideas of this model in health intervention and persuasion is quite sparse, and the challenge remains to remind professions to apply the overall tenets of humanistic psychology, namely the dignity and worth of healthy humans and their actions (Moss, 1998)

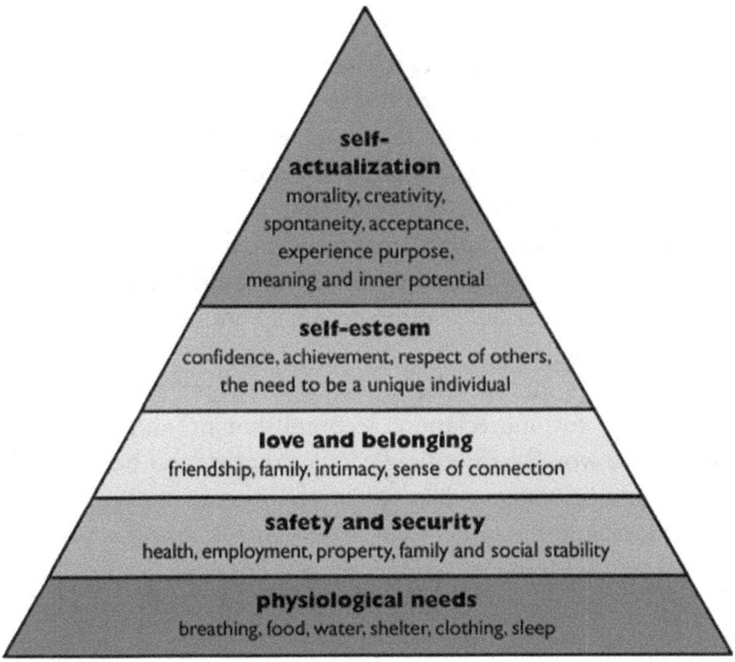

Source: https://www.researchhistory.org/2012/06/16/maslows-hierarchy-of-needs/

In the past few years, I have thought about how to best apply or include Maslow's needs levels when trying to both explain and initiate health motivation and behaviour. Despite existing criticism surrounding the alleged rigidity and linearity of explaining needs fulfilment (Wahba & Bridwell, 1976), the Maslow model follows a simple logic of how we humans evaluate and order our needs and wants. The fact that health, well-being, and safety are considered a basic need does not only explain that most of us do care for our personal and our kin's health but also that those who lack those conditions almost singularly start focusing on them. It also helps explain why people, who have a particular health condition, absorb a lot of health information and advice about how to overcome their illness and the dangers it poses—and hence can be reached easier with standard rational health communication approaches. On an aside, those individuals are also often inclined to participate in relevant research and experimental work.

Yet, for those of us who are and do feel healthy, a.k.a. have fulfilled our safety needs, the emphasis moves to the mid-tier needs of social inclusion and esteem. In other words, health if at all is not often actively thought about much, unless it contributes to achieving the fulfilment of one's social needs. Social needs, which primarily address desires such as family, community, love, inclusion, and belonging, are not only important for social development but explain an unmitigated attempt to create and preserve communal settings in one's life. One could in fact argue that we spend a vast amount of our routine personal communication to achieve and advance this need.

It is helpful to include the subsequent esteem need here, which describes a need for appreciation, accomplishment, and respect. I presume that there would be no disagreement that we feel better when our personal accomplishments, whatever they may be, are recognised and valued by our surrounding, rather than be just known to and appreciated by ourselves. The need to be valued by others is not about vanity but rather about getting a sense of our contribution to the world, which in turn increases our self-esteem and personal worth, in short adding to the formation of our self-identity and confidence. Those manifest themselves through all kinds of venues, including professional activities, science/academic achievements, arts/sports/entertainment excellence, to hobbies and random skills (think Guinness Book of Records type skills or daredevil stunts as examples for the last one).

The connection between the aforementioned and communication is motivation. It is a reason that Maslow's model has become popular in organisational and corporate leadership training. Since motivation is an intentional choice that is under the control of the person whose behaviour one aims to motivate, any leader attempting to activate self-esteem via encouraging participation needs to understand what drives the motivation to act. It is easy to see that different people are motivated by different reason or need states. It is in this field where Maslow provided not only an understanding that people differ but that motivational causes are also a moving target. Once a particular need is fulfilled it serves no longer as a cause to act. We surmise it is what makes concurrent non-communicable disease communication tricky as the targets are typically population segments who do not (believe to) have the health concern/need that a message (say, obesity prevention) is advocating. Or, if they felt to have it may have successfully overcome the biggest health consequences of the threat, and so do no longer have that concern. It is at this juncture where needs-based motivation merges with habitual behaviour.

Risk Perception, Communication, and Response

As we had previously mentioned, the phenomenon of health resistance can be understood as a lack of motivation to comply with an appeal. If we connect this with the work of scholars in humanistic psychology and neuroscience, we find that motivation to engage (or not) in some behaviour is as much habitual (reflexive, intuitive, or automatic) as it is goal-directed (i.e., a reflective or rational response).

Said simply, whereas people possess the so-called voice of reason that reminds the decision-maker to be reasonable, i.e., decide based on logical arguments, this "voice" still must do battle with people's ingrained habits and personal foibles, which create comfortable shortcuts to needs fulfilment that avoid making us think too hard whenever a decision needs to be made. In fact, most motivational decisions and modifications in our daily routines are automatic and can be triggered by seemingly random cues such as words or pictures. As we mentioned before, they happen at a level of consciousness that we often fail to explain after we engaged in the behaviour (you may have also heard of the term 'impulse buying'). So, at what category or level of health concern is a decision impulsive vs. contemplative? Or, more specifically, what drives how actual (or, shall we say, factual) health risks enter people's perceptions and assessments of them, triggering in turn a specific response?

Risk(Y) Decisions

At the time of this writing, the world has lived through a viral agent—the Severe Acute Respiratory Syndrome Corona Virus 2 (or SARS-CoV-2), leading to the disease globally known as COVID-19—that fits the technical or factual definition of a health risk, i.e., "*an event whose probability of occurring is high and whose consequences are severe in terms of direct harms, such as death, injury or environmental damage*" (Kasperson et al., 1988). Describing it further as an epidemic or pandemic, i.e., a disease outbreak that rapidly affects many people within a population, or across populations, underscores the seriousness of the risk the unassuming global population is exposed to.

This very term of 'epidemic' or 'pandemic' was however also used by popular media and public figures when describing the consequences of chosen lifestyles, e.g., overweight and obesity. We randomly grabbed a few news story headlines for illustration: (a) from the BBC—"*Obesity Pandemic*" (Walsh, 2011), (b) from NBC News—"*America's obesity epidemic, especially among women, expected to get worse*" (Edwards, 2019), (c) from the Australian ABC—"*When this community took on the obesity epidemic, it came up with 400 solutions*" (Ogilvie, 2020).

What immediately jumps out at the average critical media scholar is the position the traditional and social media are capable to occupy in skewing health perceptions and reactions. It is something that a text on communication needs to engage with, and we will do so later.

Since it is not just media writers who use vocabulary interchangeably, the other issue is whether a contagious communicable disease that is rapidly transmitted from one sufferer to others with unavoidable infections if exposed ranks factually as an equal risk to a behaviour choice that is non-communicable, speak not transferrable across people, and may or may not lead to a slow-progressing debilitation.

The fact that they still both receive the moniker of an epidemic illustrates that people have a nuanced perception of risk and related behaviours. They result from psychological, sociological, and cultural biases, such as intuition, voluntariness, economic and personal interests, ability to influence the outcome, familiarity with the hazard, size of impact, and general values held in the community (Slovic, 1987; Pidgeon et al., 2003). In other words, the precise interplay between a health risk and personal or social processes can either improve health-conducive behaviours or decrease the risk interpretation and block protective behaviours.

I have demonstrated that rational calculations and logic is not the only origin of people's decision-making. At the same token, neither is habit, intuition, or emotion. It is the constant balancing between these, often competing, interests that determine the behavioural outcome. The ratio-habit balancing act in turn is influenced by a person's socio-cultural surroundings, both structural and perceptive (peer pressures, stigmatisation, social climate) that amplify the risk response direction.

Communication Flow of Risk Messages

The communication loop model we had introduced earlier is a good basis to advance this point. The reader may remember that this model essentially explains the process of how a signal (say, a message) is moved from a sender via a channel to a receiver, undergoing an encoding process by the sender and then later a decoding one by the receiver. Please also remember that we receive dozens of 'signals' every day, some of which about the same topic (but possibly with a different content or intent).

By and large, there are two stations where a message potentially undergoes some substantial quantitative or qualitative change.

1. A receiver will use her own decoding processes and abilities (e.g., literacy, agreement, habitual patterns) to assess the message and its intent and contrast it to one's personal preferences, etc.
2. Channel entities (e.g., news media, public organisations, informal networks) can filter or alter a message during its dissemination or distribution, what Kasperson et al. (1988) called social amplification.
3. Any perceptions held about the original sender can also influence how a message is read and reacted to.

As we had mentioned in Chap. 1, persuasion scholars like Laswell (1948) and Hovland(1953) established that the average intentional message contains factual, inferential, values-based, and symbolic components. While public health puts a lot of emphasis on the information and logical conclusions that can be drawn from it, people assess those conclusions differently. They do not just use their own values constructs (e.g., 'I never get drunk after four glasses,' or 'nobody I know has suffered from this disease') but are equally attuned to the socio-cultural symbolism evoked by senders and message components. We had spoken of this when discussing health resistance in Chap. 2.

Hence, the perceived risk level of an event or action is the result of how the risk message is processed and what value is attached to it. This process routinely employs cognitive heuristics to grasp a risk's impact on one's life. For instance, the biological event of a viral agent or carcinogen invading the human cell system or the detailed effect substance abuse has on a specific organ is of little interest or concern to many, if this process is even well-comprehended. Besides its inherent complexity, a message such as this would only very circuitously make clear to the average recipient what the actual health effects are. Instead, people engage with this message selectively, and grab some rudimentary information titbits, contrasting those against known events, information, held beliefs, thoughts from trusted others, or experiences.

For COVID-19, this might invoke thought patterns like this: 'like the flu but more serious –> I had the flu before, that wasn't too serious,' 'wash hands, keep distance, wear face mask –> some say good, some say not necessary, who to believe?' 'People can die –> what people? Need to check if it is my age or area,' 'stay home –> how to make money; if I am not a target group or live in a hot spot, I can still go out, no?' 'Spreads by transmission –> can I touch this button, glass, gym equipment?' 'Get tested –> when, why, what next?' In this small hypothetical example, one can see that a lot of questions or doubts are raised as each fact is contrasted against its personal meaning and experience. And although the COVID-19 virus has spread fast and furiously, a vast majority of people have not directly experienced it or suffered from it so need to use other cues to make sense of warnings and advice. Like a product that is bought not for its functional value but for how it makes one feel so is a health risk message judged against its social or personal impact.

Factors in the Interpretation of Risk

The halo effect is a phenomenon that is part of the construction of sense-making, we explained earlier, namely that we employ prior knowledge and/or experiences along with any new objective information to form an impression of a message and its sender. If that prior perception is positive, we may give the benefit of the doubt to the new information and respond to it more positively. The halo effect has often been used to explain the role of attractiveness in producing a cognitive bias but depending on our psychological makeup, it can be other criteria (intellectual ability, charm, ruggedness, overall appearance, overlap in socio-political tendencies) that fulfill that heuristic function.

Whereas we focus on everyday people for most of the argument, it might be useful to mention that no one, including experts, are immune to it. For example, doctors may determine a patient to be healthy when that patient gives an overall impression of looking "healthy," something that only a test could verify. One can appreciate that especially for initial presentations with onset of mental health issues, which often require in-depth consultation and testing, an assessment based on the halo of a healthy appearance (assume the patient is a high-performance athlete) can lead to misdiagnoses (Gulliver et al., 2012; Hartung et al., 2010). That said, these types of misinterpretations or so-called benefits of the doubt are similarly made by lay individuals like a person's family and friends.

That the sender of most disease-prevention messages—a government department—has at best a neutral image with most people and cannot easily benefit from the pull of a halo effect from the sender. If it then must compete with more likeable senders (let's say, some internet celebrity promoting some alternative cure or protection), one can see the value of a trusted, likeable connection that spills into message decoding when required.

This is not to say that everyone employed in the health sector has a distant connection to other people. Most of us do appreciate our doctors and nurses a great deal, and this is very evident during crisis moments, where our 'first responders' and 'frontline workers' become local heroes. A sizeable number of people in any region also do work in the healthcare sector or know someone who does. It is rather that unlike these real faces of healthcare, public health divisions tasked with prevention and overall health messaging are faceless entities who are only known under their official name as National Health Department (or some such) and so are interpreted as simply the government saying something.

This goes back to what we mentioned earlier regarding the actual experience of a health risk or threat. Habit-forming—as we discussed—requires direct personal experience. So, responses by members of the public, who only encounter a health risk as a second-hand experience via information about it, its consequences and preventative management will vary along (a) any relatable life experience and (b) how the reported information is created and received. Following Kasperson et al. (1988), the latter can further be divided into four informational elements:

1. Usually, the more a health risk is mentioned (known as frequency or volume), the more people will start feeling uneasy about it. Granted, the contemporary media multitudes have created or contributed to alternative narratives on their own, even if not motivated by some ulterior motif but rather by the journalistic mantra to tell two sides of a story with only one side supported by scientific fact. However, even the most accurate or balanced coverage will struggle to assuage any fears aroused by the more frightening messages. Quoting a US scholar in paediatrics about reasoning with anti-vaccinators, "It is very easy to scare people, it is much harder to 'unscare' them" (Roehr, 2012).

Remember that we had mentioned earlier in this chapter how schemas, i.e., recollections from our past experiences help us to react swiftly to incoming information. In lack of direct experiences, these latent memories may derive from scary reports as well and prime people to assume the same about the current health crisis.

2. The idea of degrees of disagreement is really a qualitative (how the vast amount of information is communicated) extension of the first point. If key stakeholders, experts, or representative groups disagree on the facts or their inferred effects, it overall raises public concern, but it also leads to fractionalising of sub-populations along whose version one deems more credible than another's. Whereas public health issues have to date been more inoculated against the most asinine fake news and fake science critiques, they are certainly not immune to this form of debate.
3. The effect of the first two points is further enhanced when using dramatisation and sensationalist language in describing the health risk. As our brief example of calling everything an epidemic may have illustrated, media organisations in their desire to be seen by audiences as the most relevant chronicler of world events often resort to overplaying the most catastrophic consequences, spurring public fear. The above example also illustrates a persistent focus on communicable diseases even though non-communicable diseases pose the greater threat to life and livelihoods globally. Hereby, the dominant narrative that frames communicable diseases—unlike the one for non-communicable diseases—is that of a security issue, a threat that requires extraordinary responses outside of normal politics (McInnes & Roemer-Mahler, 2017; Shiffman, 2009). Aside from the media, informal communication networks with friends, relatives, or peers exist that provide reference points but also might provide cultural biases.
4. Especially those latter interactions serve to circulate and grow symbolic interpretations or associations with certain aspects of learned information. The reader may recall the argument that the routine uses of mental heuristics to engage our memories may impede the acceptance of contradictory new information to our held stereotypes or lead to memory distortion when we recall the events. These simplifications in risk assessment in, e.g., what other aspects of economic and social

life are impacted tend to become anchors for subsequent interpretations of how the health scare is managed and may become quite rigid in the face of opposing information (Chadwick, 1998; Leask et al., 2010).

Taking Advantage of Automatic Reactions

The notion of people displaying habitual reactions has been reasonably well-explained both in the academic (e.g., Kahneman, 2012) and popular (e.g., Duhigg, 2012) literature. I suspect that the reason why habits, intuitions, or emotions are not well-observed in health communication lies in the fact that they are perceived as time-consuming, unscientific, exhausting, or simply unrealistic for anyone tasked with finding a common denominator message for a large population segment.

Yet, the experience of US psychiatrist Helen Riess reveals a central insight into paying attention to them. Early in her career, Riess recognised that a real conversation (here: between doctor and patient) cannot develop if listening is just waiting for the other person to finish talking. Instead of focusing on figuring out and controlling symptoms, creating safe spaces where people felt understood and cared for reduces the emotional gap between doctor and patient (Riess, 2017; Riess et al., 2012).

One may argue that this is a scenario relevant only for such direct in-person encounters and not translatable to prevention teams. But Riess' ideas of empathy conceptually draw on both self-awareness and social awareness. The first term connects with the mental concept of self-identity, a concept that both motivates people to strive for distinctiveness and drives intergroup behaviour (Tajfel, 1974). The second term—also known as social intelligence—refers to having an in-depth understanding of societal and communal set-ups, environments, problems, struggles, norms, and cultures (Goleman, 2006; Thorndike & Lorge, 1935).

What it comes down to is an ability to understand and combine the needs of the self and others to interact in an efficient manner to deal with relevant problems and struggles for mutually beneficial outcomes. Taking a cue from management research, empathic assertiveness is comprised of the ability to emotionally relate to others' non-cognitive persona, which in turn substantially affects attitudes, reactions, and outcomes (Kellett et al., 2006).

In his 2017 witty and informative chronicle about better communication, "If I Understood You, Would I Have This Look on My Face?," Alan Alda, the award-winning actor and bestselling author, eloquently summarises what we talked about with the following rhetorical question: "*Isn't this what happens in a loving relationship when one partner helps steer the other toward his or her best instinct and values, regardless of the short-term benefits to either of them?*" (p. 144).

Epilogue

Whereas the average reflective discourse on aspects of contemporary health communication—if not exclusively a how-to manual—tends to provide problematic examples to make a case (and this one is no exception), I do not want to be remiss to add some positive habits that have impacted individuals. They are often in the form of trends or anecdotes as health entities involved with them are little inclined to call the battle won on a specific topic in fear of negating their continued existence. And it is also fanciful to assume that every single individual involved in a specific health issue will alter a habit or inclination.

That said, we have seen message-compliant behaviours improve in seatbelt use (Tison et al., 2006), dental hygiene (speak: toothbrushing) (Hobdell et al., 2003), helmet use for motor and bicycles (Heng et al., 2006:, Olivier et al., 2019), and smoking (Health Policy Analysis, 2016; West, 2017), many of which can be at least in parts traced back to new habits and emotional positions towards those behaviours. Moreover, these habit-forming trends have been shown to result from repeated focus of health communications on deeper insights into behaviours and their motivators (e.g., the national youth antismoking '*Truth*' campaign in the United States was designed to be a brand youths can identify with).

There is more to be said on the relation-forming social attentiveness approach to health communication and many of the next chapters will include further examples and ideas.

References

Alda, A. (2017). *If I understood you, would I have this look on my face?* Random House.

Andrews, B. (1903). Habit. *The American Journal of Psychology, 14*(2), 121–149.

Aue, T., Nusbaum, H., & Cacioppo, J. (2012). Neural correlates of wishful thinking. *Social Cognitive and Affective Neuroscience, 7*(8), 991–1000. https://doi.org/10.1093/scannsr081

Chadwick, P. (1998). Do media help or harm public health? *Australian and New Zealand Journal of Public Health, 22*, 155–158.

Chaiken, S., & Trope, Y. (Eds.). (1999). *Dual-process theories in social psychology*. Guilford.

Cuypers, K., Kvaløy, K., Bratberg, G., Midthjell, K., Holmen, J., & Holmen, T. (2012). Being normal weight but feeling overweight in adolescence may affect weight development into young adulthood–An 11-year follow-up: The HUNT Study, Norway. *Journal of Obesity, 2012*, 601872. https://doi.org/10.1155/2012/601872

Duhigg, C. (2012). *The power of habit: Why we do what we do and how to change*. Random House.

Edwards, E. (2019, December 19). America's obesity epidemic, especially among women, expected to get worse. *NBC Health News* https://www.nbcnews.com/health/health-news/america-s-obesity-epidemic-especially-among-women-expected-get-worse-n1103791

Epstein, S. (1991). Cognitive-experiential self-theory: An integrative theory of personality. In R. Curtis (Ed.), *The relational self: Theoretical convergences in psychoanalytical, social, and personality psychology* (pp. 111–137). Guildford.

Fazio, R. (1990). Multiple processes by which attitudes guide behavior: The MODE model as an integrative framework. In: Zanna, M. (ed.), *Advances in experimental social psychology* (Vol. 23, pp. 23–75). Academic.

Goleman, D. (2006). *Social intelligence: The new science of human relationships*. Bantam Books.

Gulliver, A., Griffiths, K., & Christensen, H. (2012). Barriers and facilitators to mental health help-seeking for young elite athletes: A qualitative study. *BMC Psychiatry, 12*, 157–171. https://doi.org/10.1186/1471-244X-12-157

Hartung, C., Lefler, E., Tempel, A., Armaendariz, M., Sigel, B., & Little, C. (2010). Halo effects in ratings of ADHD and ODD: Identification of susceptible symptoms. *Journal of Psychopathology and Behavioral Assessment, 32*, 128–137. https://doi.org/10.1007/s10862-009-9135-3

Health Policy Analysis. (2016). *Mid-point review of the National Tobacco Strategy 2012–2018: Final report*. Commonwealth Department of Health.
Heng, K., Lee, A., Zhu, S., Tham, K., & Seow, E. (2006). Helmet use and bicycle-related trauma in patients presenting to an acute hospital in Singapore. *Singapore Medical Journal, 47*(5), 367–372.
Higgs, S., & Thomas, J. (2016). Social influences on eating. *Current Opinion in Behavioral Sciences, 9*(June), 1–6.
Hobdell, M., Petersen, P., Clarkson, J., & Johnson, N. (2003). Global goals for oral health 2020. *International Dental Journal, 53*(5), 285–288. https://doi.org/10.1111/j.1875-595x.2003.tb00761.x
Hoffrage, U. (2004). Overconfidence. In R. Pohl (Ed.), *Cognitive illusions: A handbook on fallacies and biases in thinking, judgment, and memory* (pp. 235–254). Psychology Press.
Hovland, C., Janis, I., & Kelley, H. (1953). *Communication and persuasion: Psychological studies of opinion change*. Yale University Press.
Idler, E., & Kasl, S. (1995). Self-ratings of health: Do they also predict change in functional ability? *The Journals of Gerontology, 50B*(6), S344–S353. https://doi.org/10.1093/geronb/50B.6.S344
Jones, C. (2014). The Pollyanna phenomenon and non-inferiority: How our experience (and research) can lead to poor treatment choices. Science-Based Medicine. https://sciencebasedmedicine.org/the-pollyanna-phenomenon-and-non-inferiority-how-our-experience-and-research-can-lead-to-poor-treatment-choices/
Kahneman, D. (2012). *Thinking fast and slow*. Penguin Books.
Kahneman, D., & Tversky, A. (1979). Prospect theory: An analysis of decision under risk. *Econometrica, 47*(2), 263–291.
Kasperson, R., Renn, O., Slovic, P., Brown, H., Emel, J., Goble, R., Kasperson, J., & Ratick, S. (1988). The social amplification of risk: A conceptual framework. *Risk Analysis, 8*(2), 177–187.
Kellett, J., Humphrey, R., & Sleeth, R. (2006). Empathy and the emergence of task and relational leaders. *The Leadership Quarterly, 17*, 146–162.
Lasswell, H. (1948). The structure and function of communications in society. In L. Bryson (Ed.), *The communication of ideas* (pp. 37–51). Harper.
Leask, J., Hooker, C., & King, C. (2010). Media coverage of health issues and how to work more effectively with journalists: A qualitative study. *BMC Public Health, 10*, 535–542. https://doi.org/10.1186/1471-2458-10-535
Lupton, D. (2017). Digital media and body weight, shape, and size: An introduction and review. *Fat Studies, 6*(2), 119–134. https://doi.org/10.1080/21604851.2017.1243392

Major, B., Hunger, J., Bunyan, D., & Miller, C. (2014). The ironic effects of weight stigma. *Journal of Experimental Social Psychology, 51*, 74–80.

Maslow, A. (1943). A theory of human motivation. *Psychological Review, 50*(4), 370–396.

McInnes, J., & Roemer-Mahler, A. (2017). From security to risk: Reframing global health threats. *International Affairs, 93*(6), 1313–1337. https://doi.org/10.1093/ia/iix187

Merton, R. (1948). The self-fulfilling prophecy. *The Antioch Review, 8*(2), 193–210.

Moss, D. (1998). *Humanistic and transpersonal psychology: An historical and biographical sourcebook*. Greenwood.

Moss, D. (2014). The roots and genealogy of humanistic psychology. In K. Schneider, J. Pierson, & J. Bugental (Eds.), *The handbook of humanistic psychology: Theory, research, and practice* (2nd ed., pp. 3–18). Sage Publications.

Mossey, J., & Shapiro, E. (1982). Self-rated health: A predictor of mortality among the elderly. *American Journal of Public Health, 72*(8), 800–808.

Nickerson, R. (1998). Confirmation bias: A ubiquitous phenomenon in many guises. *Review of General Psychology, 2*(2), 175–220. https://doi.org/10.1037/1089-2680.2.2.175

Ogilvie, F. (2020, January 29). When this community took on the obesity epidemic, it came up with 400 solutions. *ABC News* Online. https://www.abc.net.au/news/2020-01-29/obesity-epidemic-community-based-solutions-key-to-success/11902898

Olivier, J., Boufous, S., & Grzebieta, R. (2019). The impact of bicycle helmet legislation on cycling fatalities in Australia. *International Journal of Epidemiology, 48*(4), 1197–1203.

O'Sullivan, C., & Durso, F. (1984). Effect of schema-incongruent information on memory for stereotypical attributes. *Journal of Personality and Social Psychology, 47*(1), 55–70. https://doi.org/10.1037/0022-3514.47.1.55

Petty, R., and Cacioppo, J. (1986). The elaboration likelihood model of persuasion. In: Berkowitz, L. (ed.), *Advances in experimental social psychology* (Vol. 19, pp. 123–205). Academic.

Piaget, J. (1936). *Origins of intelligence in the child*. Routledge.

Pidgeon, N., Kasperson, R., & Slovic, P. (2003). *The social amplification of risk*. Cambridge University Press.

Riess, H. (2017). The science of empathy. *Journal of Patient Experience, 4*(2), 74–77.

Riess, H., Kelley, J., Bailey, R., Dunn, E., & Phillips, M. (2012). Empathy training for resident physicians: A randomized controlled trial of a neuroscience-informed curriculum. *Journal of General Internal Medicine, 27*(10), 1280–1286. https://doi.org/10.1007/s11606-012-2063-z

Roehr, B. (2012). Media induced anti-vaccination sentiment can even affect health workers, vaccine researcher says. *BMJ, 344*(Mar01), e1563. https://doi.org/10.1136/bmj.e1563

Schwartz, A., Goldberg, J., & Hazen, G. (2008). Prospect theory, reference points, and health decisions. *Judgment and Decision making, 3*(2), 174–180.

Shiffman, J. (2009). A social explanation for the rise and fall of global health issues. *Bulletin of the World Health Organization, 87*(8), 608–613.

Slovic, P. (1987). Perception of risk. *Science, 236*, 280–290.

Smith, E., & DeCoster, J. (2000). Dual process models in social and cognitive psychology: Conceptual integration and links to underlying memory systems. *Personality and Social Psychology Review, 4*, 108–131.

Stanovich, K., West, R., & Toplak, M. (2013). Myside bias, rational thinking, and intelligence. *Current Directions in Psychological Science, 22*(4), 259–264. https://doi.org/10.1177/0963721413480174

Strack, F., & Deutsch, R. (2004). Reflective and impulsive determinants of social behavior. *Personality and Social Psychology Review, 8*(3), 220–247.

Tajfel, H. (1974). Social identity and intergroup behaviour. *Social Science Information, 13*(2), 65–93.

Thorndike, E., & Lorge, I. (1935). The influence of relevance and belonging. *Journal of Experimental Psychology, 18*, 574–584. https://doi.org/10.1037/h0063132

Tison, J., Solomon, M., Nichols, J., Gilbert, S., Siegler, J., & Cosgrove, L. (2006, May). *'Click It or Ticket' seat belt mobilization evaluation: Final report* (DOT Publication No. HS 810 979).

Tuckey, M., & Brewer, N. (2003). The influence of schemas, stimulus ambiguity, and interview schedule on eyewitness memory over time. *Journal of Experimental Psychology: Applied, 9*(2), 101–118. https://doi.org/10.1037/1076-898X.9.2.1011

Wadsworth, B. (2004). *Piaget's theory of cognitive and affective development: Foundations of constructivism*. Longman.

Wahba, M., & Bridwell, L. (1976). Maslow reconsidered: A review of research on the need hierarchy theory. *Organizational Behavior and Human Performance, 15*(2), 212–240. https://doi.org/10.1016/0030-5073(76)90038-6

Walsh, F. (2011, August 26). Obesity pandemic. *BBC News*, Health section. https://www.bbc.com/news/health-14682329

West, R. (2017). Tobacco smoking: Health impact, prevalence, correlates and interventions. *Psychology & Health, 32*(8), 1018–1036. https://doi.org/10.1080/08870446.2017.1325890

Zuckerman, M., Knee, C., Hodgins, H., & Miyake, K. (1995). Hypothesis confirmation: The joint effect of positive test strategy and acquiescence response set. *Journal of Personality and Social Psychology, 68*(1), 52–60.

4

The Politics of Talking Health: Power, Ethics, and Other Dilemmas

Overview

Medicine is an applied branch of the life (or natural) sciences, a branch that bases knowledge on observable, verifiable phenomena, or facts. Yet, what we do with those facts is deeply political. For example, determining whether pollution harms people is a matter of scientific inquiry but deciding what to do in response to those data is politics (Lopatto, 2017). Or, in health, understanding how the coronavirus infected humans and spread in their organs as well as finding a vaccine that could attack or eradicate this viral agent is a matter of scientific inquiry but deciding how we prevent a viral spread via social regulation or how to distribute a potential vaccine best and fairest was political. In short, public health—being the medical specialty primarily concerned with the promotion of health through organised efforts in society—is the part of medicine routinely exposed to and in constant communication with political matters and decisions.

Some time ago, Bambra et al. (2005) wrote a report which picked up on the argument that health and its promotion are profoundly political.

O. Werder, *Transformational Health Communication*,
https://doi.org/10.1007/978-981-99-9606-3_4

Their logical delineation of health as a commodity of influence and rights still holds true. First, like other commodities, health is regarded as a tradeable article, whose distribution and delivery are controlled or regulated by certain entities. The fact that certain socio-economic cohorts possess more of it than others or can afford to replenish it easier than others exist everywhere in the world, but the magnitude of that difference varies between societies. Next, as previously discussed, among all the areas of health that are easiest to control by political or corporate stakeholders are the environments that lead to good or bad health (known as the social determinants of health). While any action or inaction here has direct or indirect implications for the health concerns that rely on them, one should not forget that we are essentially talking about the provision of services and infrastructure in care. For example, when a government does not provide enough hospitals, low-cost/free childhood immunisations, or simply caters to economic growth ignoring traffic and pollution effects, then people's health, especially those with not enough means to seek out private solution, will suffer.

Although health and well-being had been justly included in the Universal Declaration of Human Rights (UDHR) by the United Nations General Assembly (United Nations, 1948), this has not been converted into more meaningful health discourse across the world. Although an adequate standard of health and well-being is a social right of a citizen, and it—like any other citizenship right—should experience political and social struggle to gain and secure it (Bambra et al., 2005), we are hard-pressed to find this idea of health and its political struggle as a part of public life in debates within political circles nor among society at large—unlike, say, climate change, housing, or income inequality. Aside from those debates about healthcare or coverage, health is mostly treated as 'apolitical.'

Yet, health inequalities continue to persist and sometimes even grow within and across countries, and the way governments address them lays waste to the claim of the apolitical nature of health. The fact that some societies accept health inequality as the result of individual (genetic?) differences while others seek some remedy of this 'social ill' as a necessity of a just society harks directly back to political and ideological opinions about appropriate health and social conditions. One only needs to go as far as the standard definition of ideology as a social or political philosophy, which forms the basis of economic and political theory and policy (Cranston, 2020), and we logically arrive at the notion that even the unspoken or undebated aspects of health are inherently political.

This possibly might explain why health politics, like the ongoing debate surrounding the Affordable Care Act in the United States, those surrounding the status and role of the National Health Service in the UK, or payer models of medical insurance in other countries, is so fervently focused on debates of adequate delivery of a system's healthcare and avoids a robust exchange of ideas on the right to health.

As I outlined, this stems from ideologies that dependent on whether they are of neoliberal, social democratic, libertarian, communist, or other nature situate responsibilities over a society's health to certain actors and subsequently correlate those with required services to provide adequate healthcare and products and who should offer those. In this, one can begin to spot the commodification of health or medical care (Shapiro, 2017).

Supplementing this is a particular emphasis of health (or healthy) along the biomedical meaning of *absence of disease*, something I had begun to examine in previous chapters. This restrictive definition is purposive because if the goal of health debates and decision-making is physical health, i.e., the resolution to any disease, ailment, or illness, then it logically moves services, which provide such resolution, to the fore. Not coincidentally, especially in a neoliberal economy setting, both concepts of health as commodity and health as absence of disease construct health as an individualised artefact rather than a social good and require top-down solutions from expert elites rather than the community.

Following this train of thought, if a person's health, or rather lack thereof, is the result of her personal choices and lifestyles, then each person is not only responsible for that condition but also responsible to restore her health by procuring the proper services in the healthcare marketplace (Scott-Samuel, 1979). Should these activities be insufficient to result in equal health status across the population, the best course of political action are supportive steps towards better delivery of healthcare products and services. In other words, any necessary debates in health policy need to be focused on improving or perfecting the distribution of those services by those who have the power to provide them (Marmot & Siegrist, 2010).

Undeniably, good government healthcare delivery is beneficial to a population, especially if it is well-communicated and explained. But the failure to engage in broader discussions on health and any policy and politics connected to it as an affair of the whole community not only functions as a self-fulfilling prophecy to uphold the narrow focus on care concerns as the universe of what needs to be discussed regarding health, but the exclusion of the population in this debate reduces common citizens to clients, whose main concern is to 'purchase' their way out of a state of illness back into health if required. This has two unfortunate consequences. On the one side, it shows that those who are involved in making political decisions act in quite a similar fashion than average citizens when it comes to health communication, namely choices and positions are less evidence-based but more the resultant of personal ideologies and convictions. On the other side, not being much involved in discussing health has depoliticised it for many average citizens to an extent that health behaviours may be non-compliant with campaign agendas, but they are not stemming from alternative ideas of health but rather from the resistance to authority we spoke of before. Losing—or never obtaining—a sense of ownership or autonomy over one's own health discourse is a regrettable situation, and it ought to be the role of the health communicator to remedy this dilemma or schism. Where then do the professional health communicators fit in?

A Web of Competing Interests

We occasionally hear talks about improving public's health on any topic—communicable or non-communicable—as being a "wicked problem," denoting a problem that does not have an easy solution due to incomplete, contradictory, and changing requirements (Churchman, 1967). A visiting scholar to my institute has once elegantly delineated the difference between a complicated and a complex or wicked problem with a fitting analogy. He said that a complicated problem would be like building a rocket, which seems impossible to do for the untrained person but given the parts, the time, the training, and support, we could indeed build one and shoot ourselves to the moon and back. In contrast, a complex/wicked problem would be achieving peace in the Middle East. Whichever coalition or solution one attempts, there would be some existing, shifted, or newly formed coalition, interest, or circumstance that creates the never-ending Penrose stair effect of barriers that seemingly have no real beginning or ending.

Compared with this complex example of global geopolitics, achieving a person's health seems to be a rather simple task. After all, one can justifiably argue that most people would want to be healthy for their entire life and, if this does not happen, aim to regain their health from whatever disease they are inflicted. But not unlike the analogy, there are shifting coalitions and interests at play to define a person's and a public's health and how best to address it. If excessive alcohol consumption leads to violent acts on innocents by a few, should we (a) close an entire night-time entertainment industry, (b) increase police presence, (c) staff up emergency care in nearby hospitals, (d) trust in educational approaches, or (e) prohibit alcohol distribution? If a virus threatens businesses from operating normally, do health concerns trump economic survival? These are no easy questions, and as we will discuss in a while, different jurisdictions have attempted different results.

In addition, the set of stakeholders is large and diverse. Besides the different political actors at national, regional (state, territory, province), and local levels, decisions may include medical provider organisations (both public and private), biopharma conglomerates, health insurance and other affiliated care corporations/agencies, and often non-health-related parties, who appeal for their needs. Since despite any neoliberal ideas of individual responsibility for oneself the duty for health and disease management has been largely transferred to a pool of professional and technical experts, the health provider groups have received (or taken) the power to codetermine health definitions and management affairs.

Within this contest of health policy lobbying and argumentation works the average health promotion communicator, not being a trained political actor or influencer but an expert agent or bureaucrats, who is ill-equipped (and often unwilling) to operate in the area of politicking that is foreign and often unethical to many. One anecdotal example might be a fitting stand-in for the usual disposition when things get heated.

In early 2011, the medical and health science community of Australia was alarmed about a rumoured budget cut to medical research by the then-Australian Labour government under Prime Minister Julia Gillard to the tune of up to $400 million over 4 years. In an *Australian* newspaper article, the AMA (Australian Medical Association) President Andrew Pesce was quoted to respond to this threat by saying, "*the government needs to increase the funding commitment to health and medical research to improve the evidence base, not only for cutting-edge hospital procedures but also for preventative medicine and chronic disease management*" (Dunlevy, 2011). A true statement but matter of fact with little political weight. Other interviewed leading medical scholars and practitioners at the time echoed the sentiment, also started a few petitions but overall resigned themselves to the fact that the only feasible "power" would lie in influencing what programmes could be excluded from the cuts. It is fair to add that in the end these cuts never materialised, but this was due to other actors getting involved in the political process and other priorities and constraints superseding this one.

The key insight to this anecdote revolves around the specific dilemma for public health (communication) officials. Most public health professionals tend to steer clear of the opinion battlefield of the political process, which is regarded by them as unethical, tainting one's credibility as objective, impartial, rational chroniclers of evidence and best practices if engaging in it. This thinking is reinforced every time that a political powerbroker (such as the Trump White House during the COVID pandemic) openly antagonises those reporting medical facts (that may contradict one's stance), calling them partisan opinion that reveal a political motive on the side of the health expert. In an instant, the health official can go from a no-name to a villain.

I am not arguing that health communicators should start playing political games with people's health to assert and lobby for their independent position. But recoiling from getting more involved and becoming sophisticated communicators makes it easy for political or corporate influencers to exploit credibility and expertise if it lends weight to an aligned agenda (Lamberts & Grant, 2011), yet can as easily be dismissed, ignored, or vilified if it does not serve such purpose. Most shrewd political actors know well that the opposing voice is ill-inclined to persist publicly. It was the sheer magnitude of the COVID pandemic's health threats and associated adverse political fallouts if health is not restored that offered health experts a declaredly more forceful political platform and power role in many (albeit not all) countries. One hopes this will be seen as a signal by all health communicators that being directly involved in public policy decisions has benefits.

What I have presented so far makes it clear that public health officials' work is inherently intertwined with the political process. Since politics is largely defined as a "*competition for the allocation of scarce resources*," the health of the public (or, rather, the lack thereof) will be among a shifting set of competing areas of public interest that shape many policy debates in society (Silver, 2006) and inform and shape government funding allocations.

Public health (communication) officials tend to battle a curious twin dilemma surrounding trust and leadership when it comes to addressing health in the population. On the one side, assuring disease absence via commodification in the marketplace invites a plethora of other (expert) voices to the table, who not only allegedly have some skills to assure health but also a vested interest in their definition. On the other side, any prophylactic action (speak lifestyle-adjustment interventions to ward off disease in the first place) is usually associated with less crucial government health work (aside from lethal infections), and so the average person does make little distinction between skilled frontline promoters and a top minister or other politician or powerbroker debating a course of action.

As Illich (1977) argued, independent medical professions/institutions and, even more so, drug companies routinely assert their unique qualification to be responsible for health (in the sense of curing diseases). By voicing their concerns through lobbying, they can reinforce their idea of health and, along with it, determine how political it should be (or, more typically, should not be). Public health practitioners, in contrast, usually work within government or government-affiliated organisations. This diminishes their political clout in lobbying for specific public health interventions, which may not be in favour of current government positions or actions. While a government employee opposing government health policy may not quite amount to mutiny, public debates within government are perceived differently than those between government and an outside party, like a biopharma concern or private health fund.

At the same time, the average citizen does not distinguish between a government minister, who talks to the media every day, and the vast numbers of public health employees working in a distant bureaucracy, with which very few people have direct encounters. As far as the issues about agency and resistance, we raised in Chap. 2, are concerned, health communicators at any level receive the same public distrust as the more visible actors within government, whether they were involved in a final decision or not.

And so, we close the loop to the special circumstances of dealing with wicked problems. Unlike the application or prescription of medical and pharmacological breakthroughs, public health interventions often stir controversies about the legitimate role of the state vis-à-vis individual autonomy and liberty and about the scope of personal versus social responsibility (Brown, 2010), as proposed restrictions, fines, or added taxes on issues such as smoking, alcohol, seat belt and helmet use, weight control, or prevention of sexual disease transmissions face social and moral support and objections. The rapid growth of the autism myth of the childhood MMR triad vaccine (see Davidson, 2017 for a complete chronology and analysis) has been powered by an opposing social movement of strange bedfellows from the left and right of the political spectrum in their mutual distrust of government and its intention.

While the initial impact of the now discredited and retracted Wakefield article (1998) in the Lancet about the vaccination-autism connection had surprised public health officials, it does point to the importance of good communication and dialogic ability. Yet, whereas it is of utmost importance that the choice about message content and angle is a proactive one (rather than the enforced reactive messaging required to correct misperceptions in the aftermath), it opens those statements up to the influence of subjectivity and wilful decisions, based on one's beliefs about the human condition and social circumstances (e.g., the angle of communicating obesity prevention might serve here as an example). We do not deny that empirically researched data and overall health expertise come into play, they most certainly always do. But their interpretation and subsequent use in interventions amount to a socio-political act.

Let us, then, dive deeper into the communication that is involved in "*how public institutions and actors (executives, legislatures, courts, bureaucracies, sub-national governments) and stakeholders in the private and voluntary sectors (interest groups, the media) shape the formulation and implementation of policies and programs the public health field proposes and pursues*" (Brown, 2010).

The Political Nature of Health

You may ask whether we need to concern ourselves with these matters for health communication or whether this is rather a matter for the fields of (health) policy, organisational management, or government studies. If we reduce communication to its strategic and tactical process choices (behavioural theory, message creation, channel choices) of a specific health topic, then the answer would indeed be in the negative. But if you—like me—look at this as a part of a broader web that informs and defines health communication today (including what we talk about and what not or how we say what we say to who), then we need to spend some time exploring how national (and local) health promotion and disease-prevention efforts are chosen and executed. Brown (2010), who I have cited before, started his report by stating, *"[t]he public health community seldom acknowledges that its work is pervasively political, much less explores in depth how that political saturation shapes its professional life. Public health is supposedly driven by science, whereas politics turns on tainted tasks such as raising campaign funds from special interests, pandering to voters, catering to constituents, and indulging ideologies*" (p. 156).

Despite how one may regard political acts ethically, the fact remains that all of them are enacted through communication. Since public health matters are also usually group decisions, it should be obvious that the process must be a communicative practice. That said, there appears to be overall a dearth of documented research on the complex mechanisms of decision-making on public health interventions. What we do sense (and some complain about) is that the public health capacity needed for adequate response is often insufficient in many countries (Allin et al., 2004). It is fair to admit that despite a designated public government ministry, public health—unlike, say, defence or taxation—is of an intersectoral and multilevel nature, and consequently runs into competing interests. I am not aware of any country where all-encompassing health policy measures can address, let alone resolve, a health issue independently of other ministerial sectors.

For instance, the usual non-communicable disease patterns related to smoking, alcohol, and obesity do account for a substantial percentage in many countries' burden of disease statistics, but controlling behaviours leading to comorbidities require other sectors besides the health sector. Agriculture and farming (levelling subsidies), education (increasing media and overall literacy), fiscal policies (adjusting taxation and grants), urban planning (liveable spaces, traffic flow, neighbourhood safety), and law enforcement (border control to community policing) come to mind.

That does not mean, though, that health officials cannot take leadership roles. As part of government, they can initiate policies that trigger action (state level, local level, or third parties), or assist with facilitating action items that are presented by other parties. The *Health in All Policies (HiAP)* framework, emanating from the Helsinki statement at the 8th WHO Global Conference on Health Promotion (WHO, 2014), is one such attempt. It suggests for public policies across sectors to "*systematically take into account the health implications of decisions, seek synergies, and avoid harmful health impacts in order to improve population health and health equity.*" One would assume that health officials feature prominently in advancing this collaborative framework should a government decide on it.

The Australian state of South Australia is an example for a reasonably successful implementation of this framework. Since its inception in 2007, the Health in All Policies approach has evolved through phases and is now fully integrated and coordinated by a sub-committee of the South Australian Government Cabinet, called the Executive Committee of Cabinet Chief Executives Group (CEG). Moreover, a memorandum of understanding between SA Health (the South Australian Health

Department) and the Department of Premier and Cabinet[1] assures how best to support CEG to oversee programmes and "*undertake a priority setting process in the third quarter of each calendar year, for HiAP work into the following years*" (SA Health, 2020). The HiAP framework directs all branches of government to apply an impact on public health (called the Health Lens Analysis) to a wide range of social determinants of health, such as active transport, water security, digital technology, urban development, education, employment, and sustainable regional development.

For example, recognising the link between positive education outcomes and long-term health outcomes, including increased life expectancy and reduced levels of chronic disease led to a partnership between the South Australian Department of Education and Child Development (DECD) and the Department of Health and Ageing (DHA) in 2010, called the "*Family Engagement with Literacy*" project. The aim of the project was to "*raise parental engagement with literacy to improve literacy outcomes for children in the early years of schooling, and ultimately improve their health, with a particular focus on low socio-economic families*" and led to the guided generation of relevant school-based and parent resources (SA Health, 2013).

Another approach of coordinating multidisciplinary efforts is the One Health framework. It suggests collaborative interaction to attain optimal outcomes for the interconnected areas of ecosystems, animals, and people (Evans & Leighton, 2014). It is closely related to the area of planetary health, which studies the boomerang effect to human health impacts caused by human-caused disruptions of the earth's natural systems (Almada et al., 2017). Changes in population growth, land/climate use, and global movements have led to the spread of food security issues, microbial resistance patterns, and endemic and emerging zoonotic diseases (diseases that jump from animals to people). Recent examples include West Nile virus, avian influenza (bird flu), severe acute respiratory syndrome (SARS), Ebola, Zika virus, and—of course—severe acute

[1] The Department of Premier and Cabinet (DPC) is the Australian term for the state government department or agency that provides specialist policy advice and support to the work of the government's central executive office (here, assisting the state's premier and coordination of ministerial offices). In other countries, this role might be known as privy council, chancellery, prime minister's office, cabinet secretariat, or executive office.

respiratory syndrome coronavirus 2 (SARS-CoV-2), a genetic mutation of the 2013 SARS outbreak.

While the emphasis of One Health does often centre on zoonotic infectious disease-prevention, the fields of chronic disease, mental health, injury, occupational health, and non-communicable diseases equally benefit from the approach (CDC, 2018). For example, we now know that new agricultural feed and production methods (artificial feed) as well as changes in animal husbandry (replacing grazing and foraging with confined spaces) have not only caused problems for the health of the animals but via the driver of a nutritional transition in human diets has contributed to poor nutrition, obesity, and diseases such as diabetes and cardiovascular diseases in people (Silbergeld, 2019).

The Asian Partnership for Emerging Infectious Disease Research (APEIR)—which grew out of a multi-country, multi-institutional network to fight avian influenza outbreak—is an example for applying One Health principles. The network investigates issues of disease emergence, wildlife, agricultural practices, human health, economics, and policy development. It explores the roles of wild animals and the ecological features of animal agriculture in the spread of epidemics; economic, cultural, and policy influences on subsistence and commercial animal rearing and management of disease; social and economic impacts of disease and disease control; as well as improving science and policy interactions (Veterinarians without Borders, 2010). Like HiAP, successful public health interventions require that different area experts communicate, collaborate on, and coordinate activities for the welfare of human health.

Shortfalls of Monologic Communication

Although we have made the case elsewhere that not all communication is alike, it serves to reemphasise the difference between unidirectional (monologic) and bi or multidirectional (dialogic) communication. In 1950, the American journalist and anthropologist William H. Whyte discussed the failure of motivating target groups with communicative means in a *Fortune Magazine* article: "*[t]he great enemy of communication (…) is the illusion of it. We have talked enough; but we have not listened.*

And by not listening we have failed to concede the immense complexity of our society."

Dialogic communication includes the ability to stop talking and start listening. Its relevance is evidenced by two crucial ideas. One, the repetitive creation of unidirectional (usually mass-mediated) approaches are generally only noticed by those who agree with it; the rest ignore it. The aforementioned "Fighting Fat, Fighting Fit" campaign in the UK is an apt example of an obesity prevention campaign that talked to the converted. Yet, if public health campaign creators stay convinced of the rightness of their message and the wide potential coverage of their chosen media, they will continue to assume that the message has been attended to and has done its work (Marston, 1963).

Two, this attitude also provides an opening for opposing political or other non-expert actors to relegate the scientific facts, a health campaign was based on, to the realm of opinion. This, in turn, increases behaviour adoption barriers especially for those who come to the message with already existing resistance attitudes as they now find seemingly evidentiary support for their resistance in the opposing voices. In short, it opens a Pandora's box that never needed to be touched.

Like the still-ongoing vaccination resistance movement, a plethora of best practice opinions (related to mask wearing, social distancing, quarantining, testing) advocated by politicians and other agents of influence made the rounds in the socio-political COVID pandemic discourse. While ex-president Trump disparaging his chief medical scientists may probably be an uncommon phenomenon in democracies with a well-established health system, we have witnessed comparable scorn and denial of health advice in South America, across the European continent, and parts of the Middle East and Asia. In all instances, public health experts were struggling to hold their ground, be heard, and make the necessary impact to the population.

When one experiences this, one is easy to give in to assumptions of immoral/evil motives or deviant/juvenile ignorance as is the claim in every partisan debate. But in many instances the notion of balancing scarce resources or opposing outcome goals (e.g., everybody stays healthy vs. everybody has a job and money) are criteria for those opposing health advice that trump (pardon the pun) the medical science. It reaffirms the weight of personal decision criteria on public health debates. But it also reaffirms that effective communication is about more than just imparting information. It's about understanding the emotion and intentions behind the information and delivering it in a way that invites feedback, engagement, and agreement or compromise.

The Policy of Truth (a Hint of Foucault)

As we come to the end of this chapter, the term 'beauty is in the eye of the beholder' comes to mind as a metaphor for how public health and its promotion might be envisioned in the daily ups and downs of government work and politics. Like this phrase, coined by Margaret Wolfe Hungerford in her 1878 novel Molly Bawn, which expresses that not all people have the same opinions about what is attractive, so does the understanding of health and healthy behaviours depend on the 'beholder,' in our case, the health message sender as well as its recipient.

Before I continue with the reflection, please allow a brief anecdotal observation that may provide some context. Sometime during the first COVID wave in Australia (roughly around April 2020), I happened to tune in to a popular talk show on the public ABC Network, known as Q&A. In this weekly show, a rotating five–six people panel composed of politicians, civic leaders/activists, or experts, answer prepared questions read live during the telecast by audience members and the host. In that episode the questions turned to isolation and loneliness during the new COVID pandemic and federal government social distancing advice. One of the panellists, a younger woman, focused on the statements by the routinely older, white 'family man' politicians suggesting everyone should spend the upcoming Easter Holiday with their family to prevent social gatherings and travel. Responding to that advice, she mentioned that she felt completely excluded and neglected as a single adult person. In other words, the effortlessness to comply with this health behaviour was seen from a particular subjective perspective (being already surrounded by loved ones) and unthinkingly transposed to all citizens. You can probably think of your own examples where the discourse of health and prevention by decision-makers and health leaders is interwoven with personal ambition or subjective perception.

While public health is not often a 'third rail' topic in the maelstrom that is daily government politics, the Affordable Care Act (nicknamed Obamacare) in the United States would be one example where public healthcare has become that since the Nixon administration. Like a third (or high-power conductor) rail on metro and subway tracks that power the train but can electrocute someone if they step or fall on it, so does the metaphorical use of the third rail of a nation's politics describe an issue so controversial that any public official who dares to bring it up will politically pay a high price and hence aims to avoid it. We may debate whether this indeed happened to ex-president Obama, but the ferocious debates surrounding 'socialised medicine'—as the ACA is decried by its opponents—that went on long after Obama had left office does suggest that health (or healthcare) can at times be a hot button issue in a country.

If we take this a step further, we come to the realisation that larger forces are at work in such debates. Modern parliamentarians do seldomly lead on principle but rather voice the perspectives of a group or ideology, they are beholden to. It is at this juncture, where Foucauldian ideas of the modern subject, choice making vs. self-censorship and morality come into play. Looking through the Foucault-looking glass, we may argue with Coveney (1998) that government health promotion is equally productive, informing, and assisting people to be healthy, and disciplining, reminding people of the right moral course of action and reproaching them if they deviate. Undoubtedly, modern health promotion practice is in part a consequence of public-sector reform to a new public management (NPM), inspired by ideas associated with neoliberalism (Ferlie et al., 1996). Admittedly, the above primarily happened and concerns Anglophone and some non-Anglo European countries. But what this has resulted in, among service function privatisations, reshuffles, and cuts, is the shifting of the burden of care to the family and carers (Leicht et al., 2009) due to a reconstruction of the users of health services as consumers able to make informed choices between competing services provided by the market (Henderson, 2015).

It would be repetitive to revisit at length the responsibilities and role assignments in the various health systems, with which I opened this chapter. But it is important to stress that most contemporary preventative health communication campaigns are reflective of the assumption of what Rose (2000) calls "active responsible citizens," requesting from them to engage in lifestyle choices to manage risks for future well-being after having received the tools from official communicators (Murphy, 2000). This is nowhere more manifest than in non-communicable disease areas, where lifestyle choices rather than environmental risks (e.g., virus, bacteria) cause future comorbidities but where allegedly proper and early courses of action can avoid and reduce such risks.

Crotty's (1995) analysis of obesity prevention via nutrition programmes is a worthwhile study here of how an existing medical culture and assumptions about population behaviour (here eating habits) created the early quasi-authoritarian mass education approaches about proper diets and nutrition. She surmises them as lacking "*social perspective and compassion and failing to take into consideration the everyday realities of life*" (p. 1). This singular disease-focused communication approach has meanwhile been supplemented by a community-participation model that encourages mutual communication between experts and non-experts. In thus, it created the parallel existence of a medical model (Tesh, 1988) and a social (contract) model (Ashton & Seymour, 1990). The former is composed of science-driven health promotion that reveals its ideology by basing proper individual choices on their alignment with scientific fact. The main role of health promotion in this model is to point out wayward mistakes and calls for course correction. It puts an emphasis on individual action and compliance. We spoke about this earlier. The latter, on the other hand, seeks to actively engage the targeted public and considers people's circumstances. In this approach, health promotion interventions are composed of a variety of activities, such as education, community development, and partnership with health professionals. In thus, it engages in a so-called *social contract* with its target groups and fulfilment agents (Ashton & Seymour, 1990).

Despite these apparent differences, Coveney (1998) illustrates along the example of obesity prevention that there are striking similarities between those approaches. In both instances, a self-reflective subject is required. In the medical model reflection happens because of rational engagement with scientific fact. In the contract model, it is the participation in community action after having understood social or economic constraints as the barrier to better health. To apply this to nutrition promotion, the content or involvement differs. One can talk about caloric intakes or other health hazards from repeated consumption of unhealthy foods, or one can talk about or work towards the removal of misleading advertising, lack of health food availabilities or affordability, and some such. But promotion and health experts would hardly agree to an individual's or a community's wish to eat more burgers, pizza, or candy. In either case, competence and decision-making ability—whether it is a single person's or a community of some sort—would be questioned and challenged, a principled position that was known as "*promotionism*" (Whitelaw & Whitelaw, 1996), and what Foucault termed "*pastoral power*" (Foucault, 1982).

So, this is then where Foucault enters the picture again as he was interested how a social issue and its circumstances can be made into a problem. In the case of obesity, especially childhood obesity, it was not just the alarmist nature, in which the media have created a moral panic around obesity (Campos et al., 2006), effectively coining the idea of an epidemic. The use of the BMI (Body Mass Index) as the central classification scheme used by experts to quantify healthy and unhealthy weight has added a form of identification, norming, and regulation of a seemingly at-risk physique that operates equally on the individual (disciplining the body) and community/population level (establishing problem groups and surveying them) (Evans & Colls, 2009). Resulting government strategies subsequently promote "*education for self-management as well as surveillance, reflecting a tension between the construction of children as 'active citizens' or as a vulnerable population*" (Henderson, 2015).

Foucault considered this a winning formula for official entities as "*power is exercised continuously and for what turns out to be a minimal cost*" (Foucault, 1980, p. 155). Health promotion, or all official, government-created health communication, thus creates regulation at a distance by ensuring that no matter what angle is chosen, the (target) public is tuned into the language of expertise while they are assured of their freedom and autonomy (Rose, 1990). Health communication—whether it be individually or socially oriented—provides an ethics or a means by which message recipients can assess their desires, attitudes, and conducts in relation to those set out by expertise (Coveney, 1998).

This is replicated and usually multiplied every time an infectious disease breaks out somewhere in the world. Government and health officials' responses to disease threats, such as the 2014–16 Ebola outbreak in West Africa, the 2015–16 Zika epidemic in South America, and—of course—the most recent COVID-19 global pandemic that started in 2020, have revealed both a communication battle against fear, misinformation and overreaction, and voter-motivated political behaviour that not only supported drastic and ill-conceived measures but also conflated and refocused health policy discussions about a disease with unrelated social issues (e.g., poverty/labour, immigration, race, etc.) both on a domestic as well as international scale. With public health being largely the responsibility of government public health agencies, it reveals how the state—especially in liberal democracies—can and often does exercise control over, or governs, the populace, touching on ideas of citizenship and personal responsibility for health and well-being. At the same token, it shows an official health communicator group that often struggles to produce ideology-free but convincing and motivating messages that break through an increasing clutter of voices and opinions. This in turn point to the role public health communication plays in the struggle over knowledge and power.

It is important to see how politics impacts the lives of persons around the world, including those tasked with creating health interventions. Those will logically differ depending on the country and political system one lives in. Depending on whether you are born in Canada, Portugal, China, or Pakistan, different options are available to you. And those having to address global issues, such as the WHO, need to be aware of this and navigate differences delicately but effectively. We may recall our introductory quote from Bambra et al. (2005) about health, and its promotion, being political, rendering health as a commodity of influence and rights.

As I end this chapter, I trust that nobody misunderstands its intent. It is neither meant to be raw criticism of an alleged ideological system nor is it suggesting a surrender of the purposeful work that is done in the field. On the contrary, I hope to instil a deeper reflection, debate, and possibly rejuvenation of health communication efforts for whatever health concern needs addressing. Whereas a host of commercial or semi-private entities get at times involved in the cause (e.g., in 2021 a largely anonymous medley of corporations and endowed private individuals had created a quasi-lottery, promising a lucky citizen of New South Wales one million dollars for getting fully vaccinated; and this was in fact paid out in early November), the task falls routinely to public officials. Those are by default impacted by competing action as well as politics. Remembering both the powers and fallibility of politics, it is up to the health communicator to engage in the trade unaffected by ideology and with little reliance on sheer medical evidence and a drive to fall back into top-down education. If that can be achieved, health promotion and communication can rely on their ethics and in doing so become transformative for both the intervention target population as well as the members of the agency tasked to produce health outcomes.

References

Allin, S., Mossialos, E., McKee, M., & Holland, W. (2004). *Making decisions on public health: A review of eight countries*. Brussels, Belgium, European Observatory on Health Systems and Policies (WHO).

Almada, A., Golden, C., Osofsky, S., & Myers, S. (2017). A case for planetary Health/GeoHealth. *GeoHealth, 1*(2), 75–78.

Ashton, J., & Seymour, H. (1990). *The new public health*. Open University Press.

Bambra, C., Fox, D., & Scott-Samuel, A. (2005). Towards a politics of health. *Health Promotion International, 20*(2), 187–193. https://doi.org/10.1093/heapro/dah608

Brown, L. (2010). The political face of public health. *Public Health Reviews, 32*(1), 155–173.

Campos, P., Saguy, A., Ernsberger, P., Oliver, E., & Gaesser, G. (2006). The epidemiology of overweight and obesity: Public health crisis or moral panic? *International Journal of Epidemiology, 35*(1), 55–60.

Centers for Disease Control and Prevention. (2018). *One Health basics*. CDC/National Center for Emerging and Zoonotic Infectious Diseases (NCEZID). https://www.cdc.gov/onehealth/basics/index.html

Churchman, C. (1967). Wicked problems. *Management Science, 14*(4), B141–B146. https://doi.org/10.1287/mnsc.14.4.B141

Coveney, J. (1998). The government and ethics of health promotion: The importance of Michel Foucault. *Health Education Research, 13*(3), 459–468.

Cranston, M. (2020, October 27). Ideology. In *Encyclopædia britannica.* https://www.britannica.com/topic/ideology-society

Crotty, P. (1995). *Good nutrition? Fact and fashion in dietary advice.* Allen and Unwin.

Davidson, M. (2017). Vaccination as a cause of autism-myths and controversies. *Dialogues in Clinical Neuroscience, 19*(4), 403–407.

Dunlevy, S. (2011, April 5). Scientists lash out at plans to reduce funding for research. *The Australian.* https://www.theaustralian.com.au/news/health-science/scientists-lash-out-at-plans-to-reduce-funding-for-research/news-story/ca38ed574dfc1aadba1b594a56f 24f7b

Evans, B., & Colls, R. (2009). Measuring fatness, governing bodies: The spatialities of body mass index (BMI) in anti-obesity politics. *Antipode, 41*(5), 1051–1083.

Evans, B., & Leighton, F. (2014). A history of one health. *Scientific and Technical Review (Office International des Epizooties), 33*(2), 413–420.

Ferlie, E., Pettigrew, A., & Ashburner, L. (1996). *The new public management in action.* Oxford University Press.

Foucault, M. (1980). The eye of power. In C. Gordon (Ed.), *Power/knowledge: Selected interviews and other writings 1972–1977* (pp. 146–165). Pantheon Books.

Foucault, M. (1982). The subject and power. In H. Dreyfus & P. Rabinow (Eds.), *Michel Foucault: Beyond hermeneutics and structuralism* (pp. 208–226). Harvester.

Henderson, J. (2015). Michel Foucault: Governmentality, health policy and the governance of childhood obesity. In F. Collyer (Ed.), *The Palgrave handbook of social theory in Health, illness and medicine (Chap. 21).* Springer.

Illich, I. (1977). *Limits to medicine.* Penguin.

Lamberts, R., & Grant, W. (2011, April 8). Gentlemen's rules are out, scientists: It's time to unleash the beast. *The Conversation.* https://theconversation.com/gentlemens-rules-are-out-scientists-its-time-to-unleash-the-beast-729

Leicht, K., Walter, T., Sainsaulieu, I., & Davies, S. (2009). New public management and new professionalism across nations and contexts. *Current Sociology, 57*, 581–605.

Lopatto, E. (2017, April 21). Yes, science is political. *The Verge.* https://www.theverge.com/2017/1/19/14258474/trump-inauguration-science-politics-climate-change-vaccines

Marmot, M., & Siegrist, J. (2010). *Social inequalities in health: New evidence and policy implications.* Oxford University Press.

Marston, J. (1963). *The nature of public relations*. McGraw-Hill.
Murphy, E. (2000). Risk, responsibility and rhetoric in infant feeding. *Journal of Contemporary Ethnography, 29*(3), 291–325.
Rose, H. (1990). Activists, gender and the community health movement. *Health Promotion International, 5*(3), 209–218. https://doi.org/10.1093/heapro/5.3.209.
Rose, N. (2000). Community, citizenship and the third way. *American Behavioural Scientist, 43*(9), 1395–1411.
SA Health. (2013). South Australian health in all policies initiative: Case study. SA Health. https://www.sahealth.sa.gov.au/wps/wcm/connect/f31235004fe12f72b7def7f2d1e85ff8/SA+HiAP+Initiative+Case+Study-PH%26CS-HiAP-20130604.pdf?MOD=AJPERES&;CACHEID=ROOTWORKSPACE-f31235004fe12f72b7def7f2d1e85ff8-niPMMbV
SA Health. (2020). Evolution of the health in all Policies approach. SA Health. https://www.sahealth.sa.gov.au/wps/wcm/connect/public+content/sa+health+internet/about+us/about+sa+health/health+in+all+policies
Scott-Samuel A. (1979). The politics of health. *Community medicine, 1*(2), 123–126. https://doi.org/10.1007/BF02548706.
Shapiro, B. (2017, January 11). Health care is a commodity, not a right. *National Review*. https://www.nationalreview.com/2017/01/health-care-markets-government-commodity-human-right/
Silbergeld, E. K. (2019). One Health and the Agricultural Transition in Food Animal Production. *Global Transitions, 1*, 83–92. https://doi.org/10.1016/j.glt.2019.01.003.
Silver, H. (2006). Science and politics: The uneasy relationship. *Footnotes: Newsletter of the American Sociological Association, 34*(2), 1/5.
Tesh, S. (1988). *Hidden arguments: Political ideology and disease prevention policies*. Rutgers University Press.
United Nations. (1948). *Universal declaration of human rights*. General assembly resolution 217A (III), UN Doc. A/810 at 71. United Nations.
Veterinarians Without Borders. (2010). *One health for one world: A compendium of case studies*. Veterinarians without Borders/Vètèrinaires sans Frontières–Canada. https://www.vetswithoutborders.ca/images/pdfs/OHOW%20Compendium%20Case%20Studies.pdf
Wakefield, A., Murch, S., Anthony, A., et al. (1998). Ileal-lymphoid-nodular hyperplasia, non-specific colitis, and pervasive developmental disorder in children. [retracted in: Lancet. 2010;375(9713):445]. *Lancet, 351*(9103), 637–641.

Whitelaw, S., & Whitelaw, A. (1996). What do we expect from ethics in health promotion and where does Foucault fit in? *Health Education Research, 11*(3), 349–354.
Whyte, W. (1950, September). Is anybody listening?. (p. 174). Fortune Magazine/Time.
World Health Organisation. (2014). *The Helsinki statement on health in all policies*. Helsinki, Finland: 8th Global Conference on Health Promotion.

Part II

Origins of Health Communication Barriers

5

Eudaimonia: The Tricky Endeavour to Find Evidence for Well-being or Its Absence

Overview

There must have been some anticipation in the air as the World Health Organization (WHO) delegates of the first International Conference on Health Promotion met in Ottawa in November 1986. It had been 8 years since the WHO's Alma Ata conference on primary healthcare where its resulting declaration had reaffirmed health as a fundamental human right (health for all). This not only moved prevention to the fore but also redefined it as a "*state of complete physical, mental and social wellbeing, and not merely the absence of disease*" (Declaration of Alma Ata, 1978).

Since those Alma Ata days a so-called New Public Health movement had emerged that saw a central role in promotive and preventive services to address issues of equity, poverty, social structures, or structural violence (Ashton & Thurston, 2017). While there were divergent views about what precisely constitutes the New Public Health (Ashton & Seymour, 1988; Baum, 1998; Tulchinsky & Varavikova, 2010), a shared basic premise was that "*fairness and human action, including the creation of beneficent social structures, were crucial to improving the health of human*

O. Werder, *Transformational Health Communication*,
https://doi.org/10.1007/978-981-99-9606-3_5

populations" (Baum, 1998). In a way, the Alma Ata declaration had legitimised the discussion of equity and prevention and foreshadowed this movement.

In turn, expectations grew to constitute health as the physical, social, and psychological well-being of individuals and not merely the absences of disease—a definition inimical to that of the New Public Health. When the WHO's 1986 meeting presented its 'Charter for Health Promotion,' it not only moved the promotion of lifestyles conducive to health as an equal to healthcare but firmly cemented the term of well-being as the ultimate goal of health promotion.

The Search for Well-Being

Well-being is a hard concept to wrap your head around. Typing it into your favourite search engine will invariably point you to the term 'eudaimonia' as one of the origins of the term. The concept of eudaimonia is a moral happiness concept that goes back to Aristotle's Nicomachean Ethics. It literarily translates to "good spirit" (Gåvertsson, 2015), but loosely equates with "happiness" (Deci & Ryan, 2006) and "wellness" (Kraut, 2018). Eudaimonic well-being though is not so much about the so-called good life, a worry-free, comfortable existence filled with pleasure and satisfaction of desires (a.k.a., hedonism), but a virtuous striving to live a meaningful life. At first blush the two old Greek ethics terms of *eudaimonia* and *hedonia* seem to be on equal footing when it comes to their translation into happiness or well-being. But the latter is based on the pleasures one experiences, the former on the pursuit of personal fulfilment. One also does not see the word well-being used much, when talking about hedonism.

If we're honest, it would make little sense for health promotion to conceive of a hedonistic lifestyle when engaging in its practice as it would invert the idea of prevention and support. While one would be hard-pressed to find much philosophical debate of how the idea of well-being in the Ottawa Charter should be read, it is not too far-fetched to assume that it refers to the virtuous life pursuit (speak eudaimonic) idea. Alas, this is not the end of it. It does make sense to interpret well-being as a state or drive to flourish, self-actualise, and achieve happiness for oneself and one's loved ones. And public health promotion would have a role to play as personal health is typically a vital component to achieve or preserve those conditions. But opening public health up to include psychological well-being (PWB)—a concept describing an individual's emotional health and functioning (Huppert, 2009), measured along proxies such as literacy, life expectancy, or mental functioning—still leaves out the crucial notion of the person's own view on the matter, an idea known as subjective well-being (SWB).

Unsurprisingly the study of subjective well-being is spread across multiple disciplines from philosophy and psychology to human ecology, economics, and public health (Zautra & Hempel, 1984). What roughly unites them is finding answers to how people appraise their own life, current and future. This can include both cognitive reflections (work, family, neighbourhood, etc.) as well as feelings of various types (joy, contentment, anger, stress, depression) (Diener et al., 2017). Arriving at a state in one's life that a person would determine to be desirable (the personal "quality of life" definition) does include various levels of knowledge of self-identity, development of unique potentials, core beliefs, and self-concordant goals (Waterman et al., 2010). We had discussed some of this earlier when we talked about agency, habits and motivation, and their correlation to health and healthy behaviours.

In summation, psychological well-being usually consists of mastery over one's environment, personal growth, autonomy, and purpose in life (Keyes et al., 2002). Subjective well-being, on the other hand, combines cognitive ideas of what constitutes life satisfaction with affective components towards it, whereby the positive emotions (such as joy, love) ought to outweigh the negative ones (e.g., anger, anxiety), and at best, the negative ones do not exist at all (Seligman, 2011). In that, SWB and PWB are related but empirically distinct (Hausler et al., 2017; Ring et al., 2007). I invite those interested in more details to consult the cited literature as I want to come back to the connection with health communication and promotion.

Going back to the Ottawa Charter, it mentioned well-being and its presumable definition as follows (my highlights):

> *To reach a state of* ***complete physical, mental and social well-being****, an individual or group must be able* ***to identify and to realize aspirations****, to* ***satisfy needs****, and to* ***change or cope with the environment****. (…) Health is a positive concept emphasizing* ***social and personal resources****, as well as physical capacities. Therefore, health promotion is not just the responsibility of the health sector but goes* ***beyond healthy lifestyles to well-being.*** (WHO, 1986)

Continuing to read through the charter text towards action items shows a focus on beneficial or conducive policymaking, the provision of health-supportive environments (launching the vast works and discussions surrounding 'social determinants of health'), a reorientation of health services (following on from the Alma Ata principles), and the growth of community and individual skills. The skill building support though manifests itself early as the provision of information/education as well as funding. In other words, the term well-being is not further explained, as it appears implicitly understood as the resultant of improving environmental conditions (called the '*prerequisites for health*'). At best, one can glean a definition along the psychological well-being concept, especially the ideas of environmental mastery and autonomy.

Far from criticising a push towards advocacy for equity and inclusion in a 'whole system' approach, I cannot help but feel that this overlooked the individual meaning making of well-being for a person or group, especially if that person is engaging in risky practices but does not feel any impact. As Diener et al. (2017) put it, "*[m]ore experimental research is needed on interventions in which long-term positive psychological states are raised and the effects on health assessed, including in populations who are not suffering from ill-being.*" Ironically, this focus on the amorphous well-being idea as opposed to physical illness or disease has made health interventions more complicated.

While no one suggests for a health system to wait around until a population suffers physical consequences of adverse behaviour patterns, we must admit that the process of assistance with ill health was relatively straightforward. The disease was diagnosed and then treated, following the most up-to-date medical skills and technologies. Any communication connected to this (most likely between treating doctors and patients) was also linear and direct, and discourse content was clear and established. The responsibilities lied mostly with the experts in health, however one may judge this order of things.

Assuring well-being needs to make the ready assumption that what constitutes well-being for you is the same as what constitutes well-being for me, revealing a values-based origin of the term. As I hopefully have demonstrated, the idea of well-being is multidimensional and includes physical, emotional (or psychological), social, spiritual, intellectual, and economic components. The Maslow needs hierarchy, we discussed earlier, is an element of that frame of thinking, showing the complexity and shift in what people consider important. Moreover, this working definition of well-being needs to also translate into action items, which address any hypothetical lack of well-being, and do so across sectors and communities. One cannot help but suspect that this diversity of well-being is not exactly how this term is used but rather a narrower version that focuses on physical disease-prevention via the establishment of assisting services.

Finally, the shift of health promotion away from disease-prevention, control, and reduction, and towards wellness. i.e., health being an asset for everyday life, has changed one other thing: the vision of an active, participating human being. The expectation of people actively engaging in improving their health has moved much of what leads to good health or being well into the 'to-do' basket of people themselves.

Whose Well-Being Is it Anyway?

While well-being in health unlike, say, an environmental protection effort often includes a personal or introspective element, the idea of creating equitable circumstances and the mere definition of ***social*** determinants we now toss around suggests that we also (must) engage in pro-health or well-being actions for the sake of others or the larger or common good. The nebulous definition of well-being has subsequently led hereby to excesses on both ends of the spectrum. I illustrate this along a few case studies.

Cleanliness Is Next to Godliness

Following the discussion surrounding the so-called hygiene hypothesis is a fascinating read not only into immunology and microbiology but also the struggles and foibles of having to interpret for average people what the right course of action is when raising healthy children or just living disease-free in this world. First described by Strachan (1989) to connect early childhood infection incidences with allergic diseases later in life, the hygiene hypothesis has quickly become a misnomer, interpreting hygiene with personal cleanliness. To no surprise, the alleged idea that, e.g., not washing your hands religiously is good for your overall health has come under scrutiny and was subsequentially modified or rejected (Bloomfield et al., 2016; Scudellari, 2017).

The whole debate goes back to the fact that many modern chronic inflammatory disorders of the past 100 years were found to be the result of a hygiene revolution (running toilets, water treatment, indoor living) among the well-to-do in (Western) societies in the mid to late 1800s. In other words, being too clean and protected, i.e., reducing microbial exposure, changed our immune system over generations to the point that it was unable to withstand allergic, autoimmune, and inflammatory diseases (Bloomfield et al., 2006). Strachan's work, the direct link of microbial exposure (getting dirty, so to speak) and autoimmune diseases was later challenged and refined to a loss of biodiversity in one's gut, i.e., the lack of biomes (such as probiotics) that some yoghurt commercials these days advertise to provide again (Parker, 2016). In other words, modern disease burdens are as much the result of our modern diet, high in processed foods and low in fibre as they are the result of a too-sanitary lifestyle.

What this basically means is that we modern humans increasingly suffer from diseases—such as asthma, various allergic reactions (e.g., peanut allergies, hay fevers) and inflammatory bowel diseases (e.g., Crohn's disease)—that our distant ancestors, who lived in huts and caves, living off the land, were unaccustomed to. At the same time, ongoing cautions for cleanliness have led us to create a more sterile surrounding which effectively has robbed us of some of our natural defences and reduces well-being as much as it aims to create it. Yet, it simultaneously indicates the conundrum that well-being (here: cleanliness as part of overall well-being) has caused for public health.

As I reported above, the original hygiene hypothesis, i.e., the idea that reducing hygiene practices reduce the rates of autoimmune diseases, is debated. This is not so much a head-on critique as comparative studies between industrialised and developing countries do indeed show a lower incidence rate of these diseases in developing countries (ISAAC, 1998). But as we encountered, for instance, during the spread of the successive variants of COVID-19, there are other dangers lurking when hygiene is neglected. Besides exposing oneself potentially to bouts of food poisoning due to a lack of hygiene in the home kitchen (Tachè & Carpentier, 2014), a reduction of hygiene behaviours can lead to an increased risk towards infectious diseases from SARS and Ebola to the annual flu, especially among vulnerable populations (such as the elderly or immune-compromised). As the recent pandemic illustrates, hygiene is among the fundamentals to contain infections. But since cleanliness to assure well-being is difficult to define or measure directly, misunderstandings have crept up. For the COVID pandemic, this included, among others, diverse interpretations of sanitising, distancing as well as vaccine hesitancy. The anti-vaccine stance, hereby, is partially the result of beliefs in dangerous side effects but is as much the result of a growing alternative (or holistic) view of health. Whereas the scientific community tends to look down on views antithetic to modern biology, they are in no small part the consequence of scientific work in metagenomics on the role of microbiomes for health (Guttinger, 2019), speak the hygiene hypothesis.

In short, just as for the broader term 'well-being,' the vague definition of the term has created an additional burden for public health to communicate prevention messages adequately. This is hampered further by the fact that public health experts do not operate in a vacuum (or monopolistic discourse environment) but are flanked or even contested by other sources such as the media, commercial interests, and self-declared expert opinion leaders (we'll come back to the last group in the next example). This led to calls for a smarter approach to tackle both allergy and infection issues. The result was a so-called targeted hygiene framework

(Bloomfield et al., 2016). Yet, Bloomfield et al. (2016) not only suggest more consistent and simpler messages and terminology but warn us of a lack of responsible leadership for hygiene promotion:

> *Campaigns targeting food or respiratory, pet or health-care hygiene are developed by different agencies, often with conflicting messages. They also do little to address public misunderstandings about how infections are transmitted, the difference between hygiene, cleanliness and dirt, the widespread misuse of the term 'germs', and the hygiene hypothesis misnomer.* (pp. 220–1)

To confront misinformation and to openly discuss the new insights, it is suggested that communication efforts come from a larger group of experts than just those working in epidemiology, immunology, or health policy, possibly achieving joint ownership and the dominant voice on the topic. Others (Parker, 2016) suggested people attempting self-help approaches, such as stress reduction, healthy diets, exercise, and supplement intake as those are well within the control of an individual. The benefit of both ideas lies in participation and a sense of group ownership and accomplishment, something I had spoken of before as a way to accomplish health promotion goals.

Biggest Losers and Gainers

Some may remember the reality TV show 'The Biggest Loser,' which started in the United States in 2004 and ran in close to 40 countries between 2006 and 2016 at different cycles of repetition and is still on the air in some countries. While there were variations in concepts across countries, the show's main concept revolved around a contest among overweight and obese participants to lose the most weight with the winner receiving a cash price.

Whereas this TV series did not start the trend of advice and products focused on weight management and healthy bodies, it has accelerated it with themed cookbooks, fitness DVDs, food-storage options, and protein drinks. What all these weight loss and weight management 'brands' have in common is a position of change, insisting that they help people, during a time that saw obesity rates rising in many countries. But how do we know our body is no longer healthy due to weight gain?

According to the WHO (2017), overweight and obesity are defined as "abnormal or excessive fat accumulation that presents a risk to health," typically measured via the body mass index (BMI). Having accepted the BMI as the indicator for measuring overweight, looked at from a population perspective obesity prevention typically means lowering the mean BMI level and decreasing the rate at which people enter the upper end of the BMI distribution (Institute of Medicine, 2010). With over five million people dying each year because of being overweight or obese according to the global burden of disease report collected in 2019 (WHO, 2019), there is no denying that obesity can have serious health consequences. But having cemented a simple number as the key classifier of what constitutes unhealthy weight—and by extension lower (future) well-being—has created its own sets of problems. The history of the BMI illustrates the dilemma of simplifying a complex behavioural, mental, and physical relationship into a term that has both ethical concerns and has opened the playing field to other groups with alternative motives.

The body mass index was originally invented by Belgian academic Adolphe Quetelet in 1832 (then known as the Quetelet Index or the index of the average man). Quetelet, although passionate about measuring human characteristics, was not a medical scholar, but a statistician and mathematician (Tafreshi, 2022). His aim was to establish a measure to attribute average anthropometrical data (i.e., measurements of the human body) with sociological phenomena, such as social aptitudes or deviances of races. It is worth noting that (a) Quetelet derived his formula based solely on the size and measurements of French and Scottish army conscripts, speak white middle-aged men, and (b) it was never intended as a measure of individual body fat or build. It was a way of measuring populations, not individuals, designed for the purposes of statistics, not individual health (Gordon, 2019). Whereas in its time it had been abused to measure parental fitness and to justify eugenics, it did temporarily get lost to history.

But then in the early twentieth century, US life insurances began compiling actuary tables associating height and weight with life expectancy risks and hence using those to determine policy acceptance and rates.

Since in those days only well-to-do were even able to purchase such insurances, those tables were largely based on self-reports by those individuals. Subsequently, those tables were neither random nor very accurate (Pai & Paloucek, 2000). Surprisingly, by the 1950s although life insurance tables were created by sales and accounting personnel, physicians began to use insurers' rate tables as a benchmark for evaluating weight and health.

By the 1970s, a Minnesota physiologist, named Ancel Keys, became irritated that "life insurance companies were estimating people's body fat—and hence, their risk of dying—by comparing their weights with the average weights of others of the same height, age, and gender" (Callahan, 2021). So, he and a group of fellow scientists repopularised Quetelet's index in a study of over 7000 (mostly white, middle-aged) men, where they compared his simple ratio of weight by height squared (w/h^2) to other measures, such as skin calliper measurements and underwater body density (Keys et al., 1972). The index proved equal to those and far more accurate—as well as easier—than the methods used by the insurance industry. Ironically, they not only omitted Quetelet's many papers on the topic (Karasu, 2016) but moved on to rename it—the body mass index (BMI) was borne.

With an anthropological statistician's index having entered the world of individual health, it was again the United States, where it first became connected to weight management. In 1985, the U.S. National Institutes of Health (NIH) revised their definition of "obesity," tying it to individuals' BMIs (Health Implications, 1985). Thirteen years later, the NIH changed their obesity definitions to the current—much lower—thresholds, making millions of people fat overnight (Gordon, 2019). This second change opened the doors to a new public health panic—the obesity epidemic, something we still live with. Plus, having a simply computable benchmark, prevention and treatment also aligned with it, making it the goal to lower this BMI number into the normal range. To achieve this energy balance or reduction translates in practical terms to reductions or adjustments in caloric intake (healthier diets) as well as maintenance or increase in physical activity.

Yet, if we pause for a moment, we must admit that a penchant for a quick fix to determine what healthy (or being well) looks like—and how to address its absence in all aspects of human life, not just medical ones—has opened a Pandora's box that by now is hard to adjust, let alone close.

For one, despite its statistical utility, the BMI is not very useful for individual health as it cannot distinguish between fat, muscle, or bone when it comes to a person's weight. It is hence quite likely that a muscular young athlete has the same BMI as an elderly man with increased abdominal fat. Further, a 2016 study (Tomiyama et al., 2016) established that using the BMI as the main indicator of health misclassifies people. Recruiting over 40,000 participants, the study showed that over 30% of those with "normal" BMIs were cardio-metabolically unhealthy, whereas almost 50% in the overweight BMI and 29% in the obese BMI range were cardio-metabolically healthy. Finally, having used mainly white men to validate the index, the BMI ignores the different body compositions and its variations for health connections across gender, race, and ethnicity. It should be obvious that not using women and different ethnic groups in establishing a benchmark, but then applying it to them nonetheless is arbitrary at best and dangerous at worst.

An even bigger danger lies in a situation where people, who with their doctor's support or alone have reached a healthy weight, still feel they need to shed more pounds because their BMI is too high. Or alternatively, a doctor failing to probe for potentially unhealthy habits (e.g., a poor diet) just because the patient shows a normal BMI. These situations are supplemented by all the possible fat-stigma or fat-bias scenarios that exist equally across average members of the population and doctors. In short, the body mass index is one approximation to address weight that maybe has gone too far in that it forces people into simple paradigms for the sake of establishing a well-being concept.

Itself being a product of social context—and ulterior motives—it has meanwhile been adopted as a de rigueur measurement for defining a healthy weight and overall well-being in health promotion and prevention efforts. Aside from the internal flaws listed above, it sadly also short-circuits and distracts from relevant structural factors leading to poor health, such as inequality, stigmatisation, access to healthy food, or exposure to environmental toxins (Bor et al., 2017; Costa et al., 2019; Trent et al., 2019). This does not even touch upon the cottage industry that has sprung up suggesting a quick fix to a normal BMI via diets or physical exercise with at times questionable means and approaches (Jeffery, 2021; Talbot, 2022).

Asked about how to deal with weight health, UCLA's Professor of Health Psychology Dr. Janet Tomiyama—the Dr. Tomiyama from the above-cited 2016 study—responded that one ought to prioritise behaviours that are more within one's control than the body mass index, such as "*better sleep, more exercise, getting a handle on stress and eating more fruits and vegetables*" (Callahan, 2021). Alas, we sadly seem to have all become big losers after inviting a simple alleged well-being measure into the obesity debate.

Unfulfilled Promises

In his landmark text, *Valuing Health* (2015), American philosopher Daniel Hausman challenged the reigning paradigm of measurement of health by its contribution to individual well-being. In lieu, he advocates healthcare allocation as a matter of the public instead of the private value of health. In developing his argument, he questions whether well-being is measurable. Yet he does not so much focus on any methodological challenges per se but uses its non-measurability as an argument that renders well-being inadequate in forming a basis for the valuation of health—and any connected health policy and promotion efforts that this entails. In short, his main critique centres on the reliability concern of well-being measurements being able to respect individuality, while also allowing for population-level generalisations (Alexandrova, 2017).

Although not intentional, Hausman's claim is reminiscent of medical sociologist Aaron Antonovsky's work surrounding a salutogenic model to health promotion (Antonovsky, 1979). Among Antonovsky's central concerns was that health promoters despite embracing a well-being idea seem to be persistently focused on disease-prevention (the pathogenic approach) rather than embracing an overall health-furthering (or salutogenic) approach. We ought to recall that on a conceptual level, health promotion had been linked to the grand WHO vision of '*health as a state of optimal physical, mental and social well-being*' since the 1986 charter. The thinking behind this was, of course, that if people engage in health-promoting practices, a decrease in suffering and diseases would occur.

Antonovsky summarised the problem confronting health promoters succinctly in a 1992 WHO presentation (published post-mortem as a scientific paper in 1996):

> *health promoters (in this sense no different from disease preventers) have not confronted the question of the creation of appropriate social conditions which underlie or facilitate health-promotive behaviors. (...) This debate has often centered around the 'lifestyle' concept. (...) When we look closely at the concept of 'lifestyles' as it appears in the literature, however, what is found is a list of (generally well-documented) risk factors: smoking, other substance abuse, overnutrition, drunken driving, unsafe sex, exposure to injuries. We remain squarely in the realm of disease prevention.* (pp. 11–12)

One does not have to fully agree with Antonovsky's model to notice that contemporary health promotion is still largely concerned with disease-preventive efforts, mostly addressing risk factors and how to regulate behaviours surrounding those. It begs the question why a move towards a well-being affirming (or salutogenic) behaviour-guidance approach despite the 1986 declaration has not been an easy gap to bridge.

A few years ago, I came across an interesting article written by a museum curator (Gaunt, 2016) that described a pilot programme from the University of Melbourne in Australia to expose their medical students to art in a gallery and then share their personal interpretation and feelings about it as part of their patient-related skill building. The aim, as she writes, was not the usual goal in the health sciences of achieving consensus but allow for the myriads of possible meanings and reasons. This has put most students out of their comfort zone because their training in pathology, anatomy, and physiology has taught them that there is a right and wrong answer.

In fact, scores of medical and health (promotion) researchers and practitioners have grown up in a paradigm that focuses on individual prevention of the occurrence of specific diseases. It is difficult for them to easily leave these principles of reductionism and determinism. While the individual risk-based approach makes sense for a disease-focused campaign (as diseases happen to a single individual), the area of holistic human well-being typically is impacted by being applicable to general heterogeneous publics as well as nuanced social or inter and intrapersonal influences. And while healthcare professionals and promoters are increasingly expected to be fluent in culture and social issues, these competencies exceed current training under the biomedical paradigms. Logically, biomedical training focuses on individual behavioural risk factors but training to fulfil the above expectations requires a bio-psycho-social model. In other words, a well-being focus requires to train 'empathy' or an eye for what to prioritise on a human level and to translate one's diagnoses and suggestions into community-wide encouraging messages of wellness.

Critics (Moffat, 2010; Seedhouse, 1997; Vander Schnee, 2009) have argued that scientific evidence not so much drive communication but rather perform a support role for already made decisions. This raises questions regarding the role facts and evidence play in the communication surrounding health and well-being and how they become part of the fabric of discourse that drives health promotion practice and policy.

As it stands, most of the knowledge, training, and information in health promotion still centres on what causes a disease and the treatment of any conditions rather than how to communicate and understand dialogical exchanges related to it. Aside from our earlier examples, we can also cite asbestos/cancer campaigns, which usually explain and warn of the health dangers of the chemical compounds of the material, but do not suggest ways to improve life for the entire community. This traditional interaction gives prevention campaigns the appearance of top-down health educations, instructing receivers how to reduce risks in their chosen lifestyles.

As such, well-being—despite being tossed around as an expression—effectively does not receive the depth it deserves when it comes to promotion and prevention practice. It may have to do with the unclear and debated definition of what constitutes health(y). I would rank workplace well-being programmes among those that adequately transcend the narrow 'absence of disease' definition. These employer-sponsored activities can be criticised for their self-serving motive or small-scale angles (employee assistance programmes usually include things like meditation classes, exercise groups or gym access, flexible work arrangements, healthy eating coaching, etc.), but they tend to work from a definition of well-being that starts with someone's subjective feelings about it. In other words, well-being is the measure of how employees feel about themselves and their life. This not only goes beyond the physical health definition (the above absence of disease) but moves it into the subjective well-being (SWB) definition rather than a centrally defined psychological well-being (PWB). The reader may recall my earlier discussion on the differences.

The relevance of an encompassing health or well-being perspective for any individual, let alone a community of individuals, is what Antonovsky (1996) called the salutogenic approach or the use of salutary factors. So, we'll use his own words to provide an example for how this differs from the pathogenic, single disease orientation. Using diabetes as a case, he states:

> [in the pathogenic, medical model], one is running a program to prevent non-diabetics from becoming diabetics, or diabetics from getting worse from diabetes. No matter that they die of heart attacks or are killed in traffic accidents, not to speak of disregarding any overall move toward health. That's not the job of our outfit. The person is identified with the disease, which becomes the sole focus of attention.

What he critiques is the notion of only one definition of health that every health researcher and practitioner must adhere to, when in fact health/well-being is one of those abstract words, like love and beauty, that means different things to different people (Green & Tones, 2010). Mittelmark and Bull (2013) proposed to treat this debate like other scientific debates surrounding the constitution of knowledge or whether quantitative or qualitative methods make for a superior research methodology, namely exercising a pluralistic pragmatism (the objective determines the definition). However, they do raise the need for health promotion to develop an "*increased awareness about the availability and accessibility of ways in which to measure positive aspects of well-being*" as well as an enhanced respectability of using those positive well-being indicators (p. 36). Without it, we will stubbornly remain in a dichotomy between what we call something (overall well-being) and what we address with our campaigns (risk factors connected with a specific disease).

What About the Evidence?

An additional difficulty in applying the idea of well-being in health communication is found in the application of scientific facts and empirical evidence. As illustrated in Chap. 4, it is already debatable whether all health campaigns follow the rigorous script, where scientific evidence alone drives communication. It appears in many instances that evidence performs a supporting role for otherwise made decisions. As I have argued, health priority setting in health intervention choices is (and probably must be) as political as any other policy decision. For, on the face of it, it is necessary to hold some values to promote and advance anything. The main question I posed at the time is how we arrive at the values that are chosen. To recap, what role do facts and evidence play in the communication surrounding these issues and how do they become part of the fabric of discourse that drives health promotion practice and policy. I speculated that they are relegated to support values-based choices by those in charge.

The added problem here is that if disease statistics indeed determine what health risks get promoted foremost and how they get promoted, then they may play their rightful role in providing the factual backdrop for these choices. Yet, this choice making does not speak to and advance overall well-being but to the narrower idea of the disease-prevention concept.

To begin our mind experiment, let's look at the most prevalent disease burdens (or causes of death and illness) across four countries in the early 2020s (Table 5.1).

While there were some variations across those economies (and the influence of the COVID-19 pandemic was not fully captured yet), the usual—and for that matter recurring—diseases led the list. Those were comprised of cardiological, cerebrovascular, pulmonary, and skeletal diseases. To continue this mind exercise, we then need to connect these diseases with the reasons that may lead to obtaining them. While the association is logically not complete (i.e., if one starts with the disease, there are more than the listed risk factors; if one starts with a risk factor, it may lead to other diseases), we can at least arrive at a decent priority list of what behaviours ought to be addressed with prevention efforts. Those are as follows (Fig. 5.1):

Table 5.1 Biggest disease burdens 2020–2022 across four countries

USA[a]	UK[b]	Japan[c]	Australia[d]
Heart disease/attack	Heart disease/attack	Cancer (lung)	Heart disease/attack
Cancer (skin, lung, prostate)	Stroke	Heart disease/attack	Alzheimer's disease
Chronic lung disease	Diabetes	Stroke	Stroke/thrombosis
Stroke	Parkinson's disease	Chronic lung disease	Cancer (lung)
Alzheimer's disease	Alzheimer's disease	Diabetes	Chronic lung disease
Diabetes	Rheumatoid arthritis		Diabetes

[a] Xu et al. (2022)
[b] NHS Prevalence Data (2022)
[c] Institute for Health Metrics and Evaluation (2020)
[d] Australian Bureau of Statistics (2021)

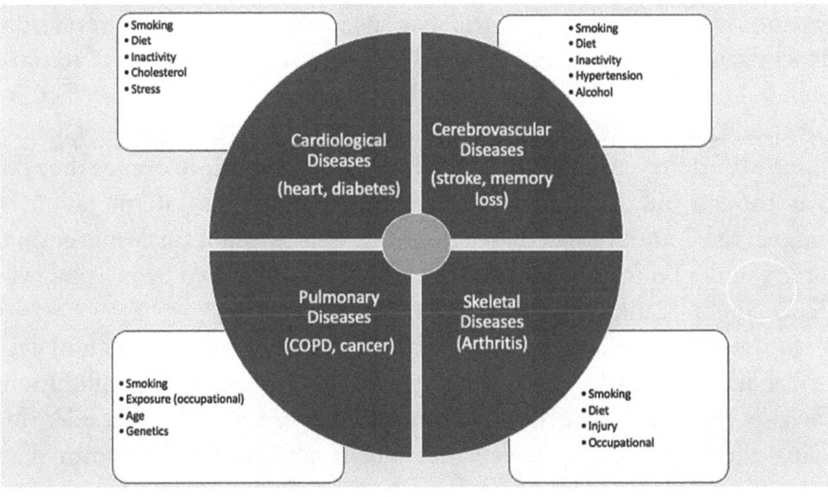

Fig. 5.1 Disease burdens and associate risk factors

We assume that those knowledgeable about public health topics (which I presume the typical reader of this book is), these connections should provide little surprise. Smoking and obesity (via diet and lack of exercise) lead the list, followed by alcohol and lifestyle or life stage influences.

Since public health efforts that aim to promote population health and well-being generally include a variety of initiatives, such as disaster preparedness, nutrition and education programmes, disease-prevention programmes, and epidemiological surveillance, it is admittedly difficult to precisely attribute national expenditures to a specific prevention campaign theme. Moreover, preventive care spending as a percentage of total health expenditures is not very high. The OECD average by 2019 was 2.4% with the UK at 3.7%, the United States at 2.9%, Japan at 2%, and Australia at 1.8% (Jackson & Shiell, 2017; Kamal & Hudman, 2020). Finally, we are well-aware and mindful that sudden health risk changes, such as the COVID-19 pandemic period, require immediate and large-scale re-allocations of efforts and spending.

That all said, two observations strike me as interesting. One, with smoking and obesity prevention efforts having this vast impact on the major lead disease burdens in many countries, one would expect for smoking and obesity campaigns to be more pronounced in terms of expenditures and share-of-voice. For instance, the tobacco prevention expenditures per capita in the past 10–15 years has fallen short of recommended levels by 70–120% depending on time frame and jurisdiction (Australian Institute of Health and Welfare, 2009; Centers for Disease Control and Prevention, 2014; WHO, 2021). Two, the relevance they do play though only reinforces the idea that well-being's interpretation is indeed risk- and disease-based as otherwise promotional prevention efforts under budgetary constraints wouldn't be as guided by medical evidence like the rankings of disease burdens as they are.

In short, we are faced by two problems. On the one side, medical evidence does not nearly dictate the choice making of and budget allocation towards prevention efforts as they may deserve. On the other side, the cause-effect relationship between risk behaviour and disease from that evidence plays too much of a role in the communicated content to have a sizeable effect on desired outcome. As an illustration, the admittedly Australia-focused ACE-Prevention (Assessing Cost Effectiveness in Prevention) report (Vos et al., 2010) is an insightful read. Evaluating the cost-effectiveness of 150 preventive health interventions, it concluded (p. 9):

- Programmes, such as Australia's skin cancer prevention, called SunSmart, need rigorous evaluation to strengthen the evidence base for its effectiveness.
- Current practice in cardiovascular prevention is inefficient.
- Most approaches promoting fruit and vegetable intake and weight loss programmes and school-based illicit drug interventions have poor cost-effectiveness credentials.
- Interventions promoting physical activity are either not well-implemented or under-funded.
- More preventive interventions for mental disorders are needed accompanied by rigorous evaluation to expand the evidence base that is still thin and short-term.
- Investments required in evaluation research to contribute to the evidence base of prevention, particularly for policy initiatives and community-based interventions that have the potential to have large health impacts but that we had to model based on suggestive rather than solid evidence. This concerns most of the population-wide taxation, regulatory and mass media interventions.

To be frank, the report also found that several of these interventions were found to improve health and reduce overall costs by securing reductions in the cost of subsequent healthcare. But while it did not (and possibly could not) provide a definitive answer—let alone one that applies to all countries—it does point to an imbalance between prevention efforts that improve health based at a reasonable cost burden based on evidence and current distribution and orientation of prevention activities.

Nutbeam (1999) argued that providing evidence that is relevant for contemporary health promotion is complex and prone to reductionist activities down the road. I believe it is where all the issues mentioned so far converge. Unlike clinical care practice, health promotion actions are more multi-faceted, which makes it harder to not only define and measure what is effective, but how to conceptualise the correct health behaviour or community well-being. This is compounded by (a) someone trained in a singular explanation overseeing these efforts and (b) the shifting position of the state as decision-maker versus enabler of empowered community action. It leads to the usual fallback on longer-term health outcomes (reduction or elimination of risk factors to avoid or reduce disease), as those are easier to measure and explain. The problem is that the time lag between communicative intervention and outcome effect is so large that the measurement of effects lacks any practical purpose.

More immediate measures, such as knowledge gain and skill building, change in social norms, and community mobilisation are so far not well-connected to the health outcomes themselves and hence open innovative communication efforts up for debate whether they achieve the longer-term goals. To truly accept the idea of good health as an essential self-determined and co-produced right of holistic health maintenance and protection rather than a person's unquestioned acceptance and adoption of the imperatives issued from the state and other health-related agencies requires more democratisation in health discourse and participation in those discourses from heretofore passive and at times resisting publics.

Since studies in health policy and health economics have found that ineffective or vacillating policymaking and the way a society is organised through these policies has an important role in health (Buchanan, 2006; Franco et al., 2004; Safael, 2006; Scott-Samuel & Springett, 2007), we should expect some effects of democratisation in health discourse interactions and participation in those discourses from so far passive and resisting publics is evident.

We know from many other fields and sectors that simple evidence-based cause-effect arguments can run into all kinds of barriers besides lack of understanding (literacy problems). The following classic joke illustrates this problem:

> *A man, who tried to win a debate, decided to use facts and evidence in his arguments. He called upon the wisdom of the ancients and reorganised it into a format that was easily digestible, tailor-made for the current audience. He pointed out every hole in his opponent's argument. His argument was logical, rational, factual.*
>
> *The second man was called on to speak. He pointed out that the first man was ugly. Then he pointed out that only 'dumb people would be on the side of the ugly man.' 'Smart people support the 2nd man's side!' When the time came to vote, the second man won in a landslide.*

I hold that a good start might be the merger of epidemiological, behavioural, cultural, and sociological research and thinking to show connections between short-term, social impacts and long-term health impacts. Moreover, successful implementations require both public awareness and political willingness for a need for action as well as a deeper understanding of the benefits vs. barriers interpretation of programmes from the perspective of a targeted public. Besides the greater inclusion of diverse stakeholders, better communication training of personnel, patience to sustain efforts, and greater sophistication in designing efforts that can break through the clutter are needed. This points to the advantage to combine different and multi-faceted intervention executions that better surround a targeted group and suggest a true care for someone's overall well-being.

References

Alexandrova, A. (2017). Is well-being measurable after all? *Public Health Ethics, 10*(2), 129–137. https://doi.org/10.1093/phe/phw015

Antonovsky, A. (1979). *Health, stress and coping*. Jossey-Bass.

Antonovsky, A. (1996). The salutogenic model as a theory to guide health promotion. *Health Promotion International, 11*(1), 11–18.

Ashton, J., & Seymour, H. (1988). *The new public health*. Open University Press.

Ashton, J., & Thurston, M. (2017). New public health. In Quah, S. (Ed.), *International Encyclopedia of Public Health* (Second Edition), (pp 231–239). Amsterdam, NL: Elsevier.

Australian Bureau of Statistics. (2021). Causes of Death, Australia. ABS. https://www.abs.gov.au/statistics/health/causes-death/causes-death-australia/2021.

Australian Institute of Health and Welfare. (2009). *Public health expenditure in Australia, 2007–08*. Health and Welfare Expenditure Series no. 38, Cat. no. HWE 47. Australian Institute of Health and Welfare. https://www.aihw.gov.au/reports/health-welfare-expenditure/health-expenditure-australia-2007-08/contents/table-of-contents

Baum, F. (1998). *The new public health of Australian perspective*. Oxford University Press.

Bloomfield, S. F., Stanwell-Smith, R., Crevel, R. W., & Pickup, J. (2006). Too clean, or not too clean: the hygiene hypothesis and home hygiene. *Clinical and experimental allergy: Journal of the British Society for Allergy and Clinical Immunology, 36*(4), 402–425. https://doi.org/10.1111/j.1365-2222.2006.02463.x.

Bloomfield, S., Rook, G. A. W., Scott, E. A., Shanahan, F., Stanwell-Smith, R., & Turner, P. (2016). Time to abandon the hygiene hypothesis: New perspectives on allergic disease, the human microbiome, infectious disease prevention and the role of targeted hygiene. *Perspectives in Public Health, 136*(4), 213–224.

Bor, J., Cohen, G., & Galea, S. (2017). Population health in an era of rising income inequality: USA, 1980–2015. *Lancet, 389*(10077), 1475–1490. https://doi.org/10.1016/S0140-6736(17)30571-8

Buchanan, D. (2006). Moral reasoning as a model for health promotion. *Social Science & Medicine, 63*, 2715–2726.

Callahan, A. (2021, May 18). Is B.M.I. A scam? *The New York Times*. https://www.nytimes.com/2021/05/18/style/is-bmi-a-scam.html

Centers for Disease Control and Prevention. (2014). *Best practices for comprehensive tobacco control programs – 2014*. United States Department of Health and Human Services, Centers for Disease Control and Prevention, Office on Smoking and Health.

Costa, B., Menezes, M., Oliveira, C., et al. (2019). Does access to healthy food vary according to socioeconomic status and to food store type? An ecologic study. *BMC Public Health, 19*, 775–780. https://doi.org/10.1186/s12889-019-6975-y

Deci, E., & Ryan, R. (2006). Self-regulation and the problem of human autonomy: Does psychology need choice, self-determination, and will? *Journal of Personality, 74*(6), 1557–1585.

Declaration of Alma-Ata International Conference on Primary Health Care, Alma-Ata, USSR. (1978), September 6–12). *Development, 47*: 159–161 (2004). https://doi.org/10.1057/palgrave.development.1100047

Diener, E., Pressman, S., Hunter, J., & Delgadillo-Chase, D. (2017). If, why, and when subjective well-being influences health, and future needed research. *Applied Psychology: Health and Well-Being, 9*, 133–167. https://doi.org/10.1111/aphw.12090

Franco, Á., Álvarez-Dardet, C., & Ruiz, M. (2004). Effect of democracy on health: Ecological study. *British Medical Journal, 329*(7480), 1421–1423.

Gaunt, H. (2016, Dec 16). Friday essay: Can looking at art make for better doctors? *The Conversation*. https://theconversation.com/friday-essay-can-looking-at-art-make-for-better-doctors-70484

Gåvertsson, F. (2015, June 12–14). *Can eudaimonism serve as a framework for a theory of rights?* Swedish Philosophy Conference, Linköping, Sweden.

Gordon, A. (2019). The bizarre and racist history of the BMI. *Elemental – A Medium Publication* (online). https://elemental.medium.com/the-bizarre-and-racist-history-of-the-bmi-7d8dc2aa33bb

Green, J., & Tones, K. (2010). *Health promotion: Planning and strategies* (2nd ed.). SAGE.

Guttinger, S. (2019). The anti-vaccination debate and the microbiome. *EMBO Reports, 20*(3), e47709. https://doi.org/10.15252/embr.201947709

Hausler, M., Strecker, C., Huber, A., Brenner, M., Höge, T., & Höfer, S. (2017). Distinguishing relational aspects of character strengths with subjective and psychological well-being. *Frontiers in Psychology, 8*, 1159–1171. https://doi.org/10.3389/fpsyg.2017.01159

Hausman, D. (2015). *Valuing health: Well-being, freedom, and suffering*. Oxford University Press.

Health Implications of Obesity. (1985). United States: U.S. Department of Health and Human Services, Public Health Service, *National Institutes of Health*, Office of Medical Applications of Research.

Huppert, F. (2009). Psychological well-being: Evidence regarding its causes and consequences. *Applied Psychology: Health and Well-Being, 1*, 137–164. https://doi.org/10.1111/j.1758-0854.2009.01008.x

Institute of Medicine (US) Committee on an Evidence Framework for Obesity Prevention Decision Making. (2010). In S. Kumanyika, L. Parker, & L. Sim (Eds.), *Bridging the evidence gap in obesity prevention: A framework to inform decision making*. National Academies Press.

Institute for Health Metrics and Evaluation (2020). Japan 2019 - What causes the most deaths? Seattle, WA: IHME. https://www.healthdata.org/research-analysis/health-bylocation/profiles/japan

ISAAC. (1998). Worldwide variation in prevalence of symptoms of asthma, allergic rhinoconjunctivitis, and atopic eczema: ISAAC. The International Study of Asthma and Allergies in Childhood (ISAAC) Steering Committee. *Lancet, 351*, 1225–1232.

Jackson, H., & Shiell, A. (2017). *Preventive health: How much does Australia spend and is it enough?* Foundation for Alcohol Research and Education.

Jeffery, Y. (2021, September 15). Diet culture is everywhere. Here's how not to buy into it. ABC Everyday Blog. https://www.abc.net.au/everyday/what-is-diet-culture-how-it-impacts-us/100291244

Kamal, R., & Hudman, J. (2020). *What do we know about spending related to public health in the U.S. and comparable countries?* Peterson KFF Health Tracker. https://www.healthsystemtracker.org/chart-collection/what-do-we-know-about-spending-related-to-public-health-in-the-u-s-and-comparable-countries/#Preventive%20care%20spending%20by%20government/compulsory%20schemes%20as%20a%20share%20of%20total%20national%20health%20expenditures,%202018

Karasu, S. (2016, March 18). Adolphe Quetelet and the evolution of body mass index (BMI). Blog Post. *Psychology Today*. https://www.psychologytoday.com/us/blog/the-gravity-weight/201603/adolphe-quetelet-and-the-evolution-body-mass-index-bmi

Keyes, C., Shmotkin, D., & Ryff, C. (2002). Optimizing well-being: The empirical encounter of two traditions. *Journal of Personal Social Psychology, 82*(6), 1007–1022. https://doi.org/10.1037/0022-3514.82.6.1007

Keys, A., Fidanza, F., Karvonen, M., Kimura, N., & Taylor, H. (1972). Indices of relative weight and obesity. *Journal of Chronic Diseases, 25*(1), 329–343. https://doi.org/10.1016/0021-9681(72)90027-6

Kraut, R. (2018). *The quality of life: Aristotle revised.* Oxford University Press.

Mittelmark, M., & Bull, T. (2013). The salutogenic model of health in health promotion research. *Global Health Promotion, 20*(2), 30–38. https://doi.org/10.1177/1757975913486684

Moffat, T. (2010). The childhood obesity epidemic: Health crisis or social construction? *Medical Anthropology Quarterly, 24*(1), 1–21.

National Health Services (2022, Dec 15). *Health Survey for England, 2021.* London, UK: NHS Digital Publication. https://digital.nhs.uk/data-andinformation/publications/statistical/health-survey-for-england/2021.

Nutbeam, D. (1999). The challenge to provide evidence in health promotion. *Health Promotion International, 14*(2), 99–101.

Pai, M., & Paloucek, F. (2000). The origin of the "ideal" body weight equations. *Annals of Pharmacotherapy, 34*(9), 1066–1069. https://doi.org/10.1345/aph.19381

Parker, W. (2016, January 13). If being too clean makes us sick, why isn't getting dirty the solution? *The Conversation.* https://theconversation.com/if-being-too-clean-makes-us-sick-why-isnt-getting-dirty-the-solution-50572

Ring, L., Höfer, S., McGee, H., Hickey, A., & O'Boyle, C. (2007). Individual quality of life: Can it be accounted for by psychological or subjective well-being? *Social Indicators Research, 82*, 443–461. https://doi.org/10.1007/s11205-006-9041-y

Safael, J. (2006). Is democracy good for health? *International Journal of Health Services, 36*(4), 767–786.

Scott-Samuel, A., & Springett, J. (2007). Hegemony or health promotion? Prospects for reviving England's lost discipline. *Journal of the Royal Society for the Promotion of Health, 127*(5), 211–214.

Scudellari, M. (2017). News feature: Cleaning up the hygiene hypothesis. *Proceedings of the National Academy of Sciences of the United States of America, 114*(7), 1433–1436.

Seedhouse, D. (1997). *Health promotion: Philosophy, prejudice and practice.* Wiley.

Seligman, M. (2011). *Flourish: A visionary new understanding of happiness and well-being.* Free Press.

Strachan, D. (1989). Hay fever, hygiene, and household size. *British Medical Journal (Clinical Research ed.), 299*(6710), 1259–1260. https://doi.org/10.1136/bmj.299.6710.1259

Tachè, B., & Carpentier, B. (2014). Hygiene in the home kitchen: Changes in behaviour and impact of key microbiological hazard control measures. *Food Control, 35*(1), 392–400.

Tafreshi, D. (2022). Adolphe Quetelet and the legacy of the "average man" in psychology. *Historical of Psychology, 25*(1), 34–55. https://doi.org/10.1037/hop0000202

Talbot, M. (2022, March 21). Exercise is good for you. The exercise industry may not be. *The New Yorker.* https://www.newyorker.com/magazine/2022/03/21/exercise-is-good-for-you-the-exercise-industry-may-not-be

Tomiyama, A., Hunger, J., Nguyen-Cuu, J., & Wells, C. (2016). Misclassification of cardiometabolic health when using body mass index categories in NHANES 2005–2012. *International Journal of Obesity, 40,* 8830886. https://doi.org/10.1038/ijo.2016.17

Trent, M., Dooley, D., Dougè, J., et al. (2019). Section on adolescent health; council on community Pediatrics; committee on adolescence. The impact of racism on child and adolescent health. *Pediatrics, 144*(2), e20191765. https://doi.org/10.1542/peds.2019-1765

Tulchinsky, T., & Varavikova, E. (2010). What is the "new public health"? *Public Health Reviews, 32,* 25–53. https://doi.org/10.1007/BF03391592

Vander Schnee, J. (2009). Fruit, vegetables, fatness and Foucault: Governing students and their families through health policy. *Journal of Education Policy, 24*(5), 557–574.

Vos, T., Carter, R., Barendregt, J., Mihalopoulos, C., Veerman, L., Magnus, A., Cobiac, L., Bertram, M., & Wallace, A. (2010). *Assessing cost-effectiveness in prevention (ACE–prevention): Final report.* University of Queensland and Deakin University.

Waterman, A., Schwartz, S., Zamboanga, B., Ravert, R., Williams, M., Bede Agocha, V., et al. (2010). The questionnaire for eudaimonic well-being:

Psychometric properties, demographic comparisons, and evidence of validity. *Journal of Positive Psychology, 5*(1), 41–61.
World Health Organisation. (1986). *Ottawa charter for health promotion: First international conference on health promotion, Ottawa, 21 November 1986.* WHO. https://www.healthpromotion.org.au/images/ottawa_charter_hp.pdf
World Health Organisation. (2019). *Fact sheet: Obesity*. WHO. https://www.who.int/news-room/fact-sheets/detail/obesity-and-overweight
World Health Organisation. (2021). *It's time to invest in cessation: The global investment case for tobacco cessation.* WHO. https://www.who.int/publications/i/item/9789240039308
Xu, J., Murphy, S., Kochanek, K., & Arias, E. (2022). Mortality in the United States, 2021. National Center for Health Statistics Data Brief No. 456, December 2022. Atlanta, GA: CDC.
Zautra, A., & Hempel, A. (1984). Subjective well-being and physical health: A narrative literature review with suggestions for future research. *The International Journal of Aging and Human Development, 19*(2), 95–110.

6

Culture's Consequences: Making Health Communication More Equitable and Inclusive

Overview

In 2008 the World Health Organization (2008) identified housing, employment conditions, education, social relationships, income, poverty, and the distribution of power and resources as key factors for ill health or its prevention. These are, of course, the well-known social determinants of health, which constitute a way of thinking about the causes of healthy or unhealthy behaviours, and an angle to use for promotional activities and intervention campaigns. Notably absent in the original list is culture. Whenever it is mentioned as a determinant—typically when discussing Indigenous or minority group health—it is framed as a problem, rather than a basis for opportunities (George et al., 2019). 'Culture' is reinterpreted as a contributing factor to risky behaviours, e.g., in matters of drug and alcohol use. What is precisely meant by culture in that context is not very clear and it appears to be used as a placeholder for race (Bond et al., 2021), an issue that is by itself problematic.

Overall, culture does matter a great deal for all human communication and activity. All of us have been nurtured into and are perpetually impacted by a set of locally defined forms of behaviour and discourse

O. Werder, *Transformational Health Communication*,
https://doi.org/10.1007/978-981-99-9606-3_6

patterns that pertain to all aspects of our lives. As such, culture affects everything from birth to old age (e.g., education, personal daily routines, social interactions, or work), and those systems also shape how health and risk messaging is received and followed (Iwelunmor & Airhihenbuwa, 2017). In general, culture refers to the values, beliefs, attitudes, accepted actions, and general characteristics of a group of people. While we tend to think of culture in terms of national or ethnic groups, it can equally include groups based on age, religion, education, ability, gender, or income. In health communication, it is often these latter groups who are not always adequately addressed.

The omnipresence of culture dawned on me first in my undergraduate degree when we studied the work of the Dutch anthropologist Geert Hofstede in my international management and marketing course. His seminal book, *Culture's Consequences* (1980), established an efficient interpretive framework for grasping cultural differences on a global scale. The five dimensions of culture he defined—such as power distance (a culture accepts or rejects unequal power distribution) and uncertainty avoidance (a culture has high or low levels of endorsing ambiguity and risk-taking)—provided a useful guide to be mindful of how cultures differ. It is true that culture here is referring to national or pan-regional properties, but the dimensions nonetheless provided a better grasp of culture's effects.

What it did for the world of international marketing and management was to transcend the surface adjustments. Where before cross-cultural promotions blunders were only recognised if they came about as badly translated or stereotyping names, slogans, or logos, it became now more nuanced, meaning that even if a campaign or marketing execution seems generic, it may still fail because a culture's values and patterns were violated. A memorable example that did pay attention to this, I recall, was the French men's cologne *Drakkar Noir* by Guy Laroche. To sell the brand in the Middle East it adapted to Muslim culture both in terms of insinuated nudity and gender relationships by completely adjusting its image (what was a naked male arm holding the fragrance bottle and being gripped by a woman's hand became a tuxedo-clad male arm holding the same bottle and being barely touched by a woman's fingernail).

Effects of Culture in Healthcare and Promotion

Although several books have meanwhile been written about the relevance of culture as a factor for health (e.g., Hsieh & Kramer, 2021; Lewis & Lewis, 2015; Zoller & Dutta, 2008), it seems to have remained more of a rhetorical debate than an applied concept in healthcare promotion practice. The same can be said for interpersonal communication, such as doctor-patient interaction, where the insight that cultural competency facilitates cross-cultural communication, which in turn improves healthcare challenges when communicating with a member from a cultural group, has not been adopted as widely as desirable.

Here are a few examples why culture matters. Research into the interplay of cultural values of Muslims and doctor-patient engagement has revealed that the Islamic faith can influence health practices, risks, and the use of healthcare as much as everyday decision-making and family dynamics (Mutair et al., 2014). For example, male doctors at times need to communicate through a spouse if the patient is female. If in that instance "*a male healthcare professional is talking to or asking questions of a female patient while her partner is in the room, but the patient does not respond, the healthcare professional should ask the patient if she would prefer, he talk to the partner*" (Attum et al., 2023). Otherwise, he will not make any progress in that conversation.

Among immigrants in Australia, similar to immigrants in other Western countries, there is a delay in health-seeking and poor uptake of screening. While social determinants (limited mobility, work schedules, lack of interpreter services) play a role, especially migrant women perceive a gap between the medical advice they are given and their own health beliefs and concepts of good treatment. They share their experiences to other community members creating a subjective perception of the host country's services that, in turn, also reveals the migrant culture's community values, healthcare expectations, and social relationships (Manderson & Allotey, 2003). I became personally aware of those barriers when being involved for a time with pre-diabetes and diabetes prevention efforts in a part of Sydney that has a proportionally high immigrant population from South Asia. Prevention services and even doctor visits had been lacking by members of those communities until a culturally more inclusive information and motivation campaign (including, among others, public events that involved entertainers from those countries) was launched.

Relatedly, some years before, I was involved with a research group in the US-state of New Mexico on improving the promotion of a mobile mammography lab (in essence, a van or overland bus with a screening device in the back, which offers free breast cancer screening) that travels to the rural and native American population in the remote parts of the state. The target groups, composed mostly of middle-aged to older women of rural Latina (largely Mexican origin) and resident Native American tribal (predominantly Navajo and Pueblo tribes) women of the same age ranges, seemed to use this free service far less than expected. Once again, the original idea for that service had taken the most relevant social determinants into consideration by offering a solution to (a) too great a distance to an equipped medical facility and (b) lack of knowledge of how to avoid the most severe consequences of this cancer. What was neglected were cultural barriers to participation, namely cultural morals, and attitudes towards the procedure, such as exposing one's breasts to a stranger, a mistrust in a machine being better than the local healer or trusted alternative medicine provider, and an overall scepticism of the motives of an Anglo-White government health service team rolling into town when typically, it is overlooked and forgotten.

Culture, as I mentioned above, also does not just pertain to national or ethnic differences. For instance, beliefs about masculinity and manhood that are deeply rooted in culture play a role in shaping the behavioural patterns of men in ways that have consequences for health. Men in many countries are socialised to project strength, individuality, autonomy, dominance, stoicism, and physical aggression, and to avoid demonstrations of emotion or vulnerability that could be construed as weakness (Williams, 2003). These customs often translate into fewer encounters with the healthcare system, delayed attention to symptoms, poor medication compliance, and an unwillingness to talk openly about health concerns (Liburd et al., 2007), which has particularly become a problem in recent years for the growing necessity of mental health early intervention.

In all these examples, it shows the effect that culture has on someone's behaviour. Since the objective of health communication is behaviour or lifestyle modification, it is worth to highlight again that lifestyle practices cannot be addressed independently from people's cultural backgrounds. But I need to equally reemphasise the cultural restraints of those tasked with research or campaign executions addressed at a cultural group from a different background. They too hail from a particular culture that takes certain reactions and responses for granted and often expects them to occur in a specific format foreign to culturally distant groups. Published health promotion research alone—whether academic or institutional—usually originates from investigators in high-income and western countries. Their personal cultural biases and perspectives influence their lenses of scientific inquiry (Al-Bannay et al., 2014), and, in the following, those of the practitioners exposed to those reports.

Culture-Aware Health Communication

Many health promotion strategies and programmes have failed to design programmes for populations with complex and diverse needs that reflect social and cultural realities and are meaningful to people's health practices and beliefs (Vaughn & Krenz, 2013). In fact, research in health psychology shows a growing discontent with the ambiguous results of employing the individualistic, acultural constructs of mainstream cognitive social psychology in messages and campaigns (Ford et al., 2015; Gutchess & Rajaram, 2023; Smith & Bond, 2022). As I had mentioned elsewhere, the traditional health communication paradigm omits the community-building and community-sustaining function of communication.

One shift to this paradigm was proposed by Mohan Dutta (2007) in developing a culture-centred approach (CCA) to health communication. The CCA moves health communication from the message-based behaviour approach to one of community advocacy and building communicative infrastructures. It does so by moving culture at the centre of the communication process so that any communicative outcomes (such as a health communication theory or a campaign) are contextually embedded and co-constructed through dialogue with the cultural participants. What it achieves is twofold. One, by providing and engaging with community spaces that allow members to practise their cultural resources that enable health—such as cultural artefacts, songs, art, and dance—a culture-aware approach redefines discourses about health beyond the narrow biomedical framework. And two, by highlighting the symbolic and communicative meaning of physical structural inequities (healthcare delivery, schools, neighbourhoods, childcare centres), it opens the conversation on health and healthy living (Duncan, 2017). Both seem to have a spiritual connection to a research and practice approach I will discuss in the final chapter. Health humanities aims to include overlooked stakeholders to get involved in healthcare and prevention by involving the arts and humanities, which in turn forces a rethink of how to communicate about health behaviours and services.

Another attractive way of thinking about addressing cultural effects in health communication practice is borrowing ideas from social representation (Hall, 1997; Howarth, 2011). It argues that since "*culture informs the ways we think and act in relation to everything—even the ways in which we think about communication*," communicative exchanges are deeply cultural (Porter & Samovar, 1988). On the one side, social representation offers an explanation of communication as an instrument to develop and advance shared cultural values and social practices. This helps us to understand the nature of resistance and transformation within communicative exchange (Moscovici, 1961/2008). On the other side, looking at it from the cultural studies perspective, advanced by Stuart Hall (1980), adds the political dimension of representation via communication that touches upon ideological constructions of reality by the media and other public institutions to sustain systems of power and inequality (Hall, 1997).

Although this sounds abstract, a study by Rateau et al. (2023) on the social representation of the coronavirus and its causal perceptions shows its relevance and applicability. The study found that individuals responded more positively to calls for public vaccination communications if those messages showed how vaccination reduces contagion and mortality rates as those two were listed by respondents as the central threat representations. They reacted more indifferent if arguments were based on solidarity with the most vulnerable people. Yet simultaneously, those people believing that the virus was intentionally manufactured developed a social representation that incorporated a central conspiratorial view of COVID-19, which undermined the effectiveness of any vaccination promotion campaign (pp. 108–109).

Another example of understanding shared cultural values and practices was the Truth campaign's 2015 music video, "*Left Swipe Dat*," aired during the 57th annual Grammy Awards, and featuring internet icons such as Becky G and Fifth Harmony (YouTube and social media influencers and celebrities, this audience was very familiar with). Cognisant of youth culture and its dating habits, the video calls attention to the impact of smoking images on dating success. Using the results of a social experiment on the popular dating app, Tinder, that showed that profile pictures which include images of smoking get twice as many "left swipes" or rejections as those that do not, "*Left Swipe Dat*" highlights images of smoking posted by some young people on dating platforms in a humorous approach to define smokers as unattractive (Russell, 2015).

The video has been viewed online more than 48 million times and quickly earned it a place in youth pop culture. The handle *#leftswipedat* became a number one trending topic across social platforms worldwide and the phrase "Left Swipe That" now appears in the Urban Dictionary. More importantly, it drove more than 1.9 million visits to thetruth.com website and according to media use and cohort smoking behaviour tracking studies by Truth led to significant changes in awareness and campaign related attitudes about smoking throughout the course of the campaign (truth initiative, 2015). What it also demonstrated is that harnessing cultural representations, such as media use and cultural elements and icons, in the case of youth culture consisting of popular content creators (influencers) and messages (memes) endemic to social media, is an encouraging approach to achieve better health campaign awareness and engagement (Kostygina et al., 2020).

Although not everyone was equally enthusiastic about this campaign—critiquing a dating habit that not all smoking youths share or being too flashy and creative-awards driven but less clear on achieving its end goal—what this campaign did achieve was transcending the typical idea of community and representation. When public health policymakers discuss health promotion resources for communities, they tend to refer to geographically located communities, also known as "communities of place," whereas this campaign targeted a so-called community of identity (Campbell & Murray, 2004). We can intuitively comprehend that there is a difference between a geographical locale and a widely distributed but lifestyle or behaviourally based homogeneous group. So, when health promoters look at a community as a specific place, it is in parts a matter of convenience and expedience for communication purposes. This is by itself questionable as the example above for reaching young people but also HIV/AIDS prevention campaigns that focus on a neighbourhood or specific place can attest to.

Yet, there is even a more serious problem involved as the "community of place" concept in communication outreach reveals socially constructed factors like power, exclusion, sexuality, ability, and protection of vested interests (Fremeaux, 2005; Stephens, 2007). Those were the issues addressed by Hall's political dimension of representation.

Making Health Communication More Equitable

If COVID-19 had any benefits, it might be the recognition by many health entities that their capacity and structure led to their public health guidance not having been able to reach all people equally in a timely and effective manner. As the WHO attested to in a spotlight report (2020), this was in large part the result of a lack of solidarity between nations, institutions, communities, and individuals, exacerbating already exiting "*health inequities related to income, gender, ethnicity, living in remote rural areas or disadvantaged urban areas, education, occupation/employment conditions, and disability.*"

If we—as I have attempted to do throughout this book—accept that all communication about health, whether it is a strategically targeted campaign, a socio-economic policy debate, a visit to the doctor or hospital, or four friends discussing an unhealthy habit, is a vital part in how equitable health is distributed, then we must admit that there are numerous contestations about what is the most appropriate way to address it. Since such debates are typically driven by the values of organisational, government, religious, or social power brokers, they inevitably include struggles over the social and economic structural causes of lack of health and inequality of resource provision and access. This demonstrates nothing else than that health is not just about medical and scientific breakthroughs, or individual behaviour management, but also about power and control.

Lewis and Lewis (2015) have adroitly summarised how various disenfranchised or stigmatised communities have taken matters into their own hands and employed their own modes of communication to form coalitions and alliances (such as activist groups or advocacy organisations) to correct misperceptions, provide spaces for regular citizens to reconnect and participate as well as find support, and influence decision-makers in turn. What I am most interested in with this part though is how public health promotion experts can create a basic level of trust for people to engage and participate.

From a research perspective this may be achieved when employing a methodological approach known as community-based participatory research (CBPR), which I will talk more about elsewhere. The inclusion of communities as partners can take many forms (Wallerstein et al., 2018). For example, in a research project on school-based adolescent obesity prevention, I was involved with (Sussman et al., 2013), overweight/obese adolescent and parent dyads from the targeted schools were recruited onto a community advisory council to assist with the formative assessment of potential intervention tools. To be honest, CBPR is still debated, and questions remain about whether it is feasible or useful (Saitz, 2018) in public health and health promotion research. Yet, it seems researchers are ahead of institutional promotion and care practice, where certain groups have been more systematically shut out of decision-making processes that directly impact their lives. Achieving health equity means that health status and outcomes won't be predictable based on a person's identities or characteristics (Braveman et al., 2017). For communication efforts it means, among others, to avoid unnecessary access barriers such as complex health systems and outputs.

A Word on Health Literacy

Health literacy is the term used to describe a person's ability to access, comprehend, and properly use health information and behavioural nudges. Since health literacy contributes to differences in patient/consumer knowledge, self-efficacy, self-care behaviour, and health status, individuals lacking health literacy are less able to engage in community dialogues on health and healthcare, which reduces their involvement in clinical decision-making, their inclination to bring up personal health concerns with doctors, and proper observance of treatment plans and advice (Kripalani et al., 2010; Osborn et al., 2011; Sørensen et al., 2012).

Given that low or inadequate health literacy rates are disproportionally higher among minority, migrant, rural, and low SES groups, a minimum necessity for health communication ought to be lowering barriers to access and understanding of health information for those groups. Although there have been improvements in the past decades, it is surprising how technical, legalistic, or jargon-laden many public-facing documents (e.g., health insurance forms, hospital intake sheets, medicine prescription leaflets) and officials' statements (doctors' diagnoses and treatment advice, general self-care announcements like the daily media conferences given by medical officers during the COVID pandemic) still are. Besides lacking clarity, they also often appear static, monotonous, exclusive, distant, and unrelatable. The last dot point highlights the relevance of creating material and resources that reflect someone's lived experiences so the targeted community can see itself reflected in that communication.

One possible way is to use the services of editorial or readability tools that health communicators can use to check on the understandability and actionability of their printable or audio-visual education or promotion materials. There are meanwhile a few in various stages of development or testing, such as the Patient Education Materials Assessment Tool (PEMAT) (Shoemaker et al., 2014) or the Sydney Health Literacy Lab (SHeLL) Editor (Ayre et al., 2023). Alternatively, one can outsource this work to health literacy or plain language service businesses.

Yet, besides the fact that not all communication is in the form of prepared materials, we ought to remember the cultural embeddedness of the understanding and discourse of health. That is, the meanings receivers draw from messages depend on how receivers incorporate them into their ways of understanding and everyday talk. The way people are able or prefer to acquire knowledge is based on their conventional sensemaking, how they typically talk to or consult with those with authority in their own family or community, the trust they have in health professionals, the frequency and fondness they display towards the use of technology and, of course, the influence they receive from their peer groups. Some of the strongest influences on people's health literacy development are social practices that start from early infant experiences. They include stories and myths; cultural and community practices; family, friends, and peers; the workplace; and—if regularly using the health system—health workers (WHO, 2022). Since this establishes not only the sensemaking of health content but also the health-seeking behaviour if any, to make a difference requires a direct engagement with processes in a community of interest. Depending on who that group is, it could be a women's health network, a men's sporting club, an LGBTIQ+ social group, a youth event, a country women's association, a religious network, and so on.

A Framework for Better Communication

The excursion into health literacy expounded that especially mediated health communication interventions may reinforce existing social and educational disparities. As research (Salmon et al., 1996; Viswanath et al., 1991) found, the reasons are twofold. One, compared to the disenfranchised groups we spoke of earlier in this chapter, higher SES, urban, and majority population segments tend to walk away with increased knowledge of a relevant health issue after a campaign despite equal motivation prior to the information campaign. This phenomenon is known as the knowledge gap hypothesis. It stipulates that because higher SES population segments acquire mass media information faster, using more media outlets paired with the easier access to those by higher SES groups widens the knowledge of a health topic and suggested coursed of action between those groups.

Two, health intervention recommendations are also often ignorant of the cultural or emotional significance of a deemed unhealthy practice by marginalised population groups (Guttman & Salmon, 2004). It leads to campaigns that successfully reach mostly those groups who already engage in a conducive behaviour. These are unsurprisingly typically those higher SES segments from the first point. What this requires in the first step is a more reflective preparation of a health intervention. Reflective both in terms of the knowledge and attitude towards the health issue of the intended receiver, but also the potential bias and familiarity with the target group on the side of the message sender.

A few years ago, I presented a process model of digital health communication at a communication conference that was an adaptation of the social information process model of media use (Fulk et al., 1987), and we had a lively debate whether socio-psychological models exploring attitude formation of individuals in the workplace (or comparable organisational settings) can be applied to health promotion developments. What we did agree on rapidly was that health promoters are as equally influenced by their socio-cultural embeddedness as receivers. This along with their experience in target- or culture-specific engagement (say, knowing how to create health narratives that a subgroup comprehends and associates with) changes the original objective communication task to a perceived or biased one.

There is nothing inherently dramatic about communicators becoming or being aware of their ideological predisposition and factual beliefs although those conditions will influence the message encoding process. Being clear and honest about one's own problem definition and evidence interpretation, however, allows to look at the problem from a 360-degree view, uncover possible knowledge gaps or cultural beliefs or values that interact with a suggested behaviour, and reflect on how communication or policy so far has reduced or created barriers and has assisted with being either inclusive or maintaining a status quo.

After completing this step and defining accurately the priority audience, it is time to engage with, actively listen to, and collect information/feedback from that audience in a more dialogic fashion. What I mean by meaningful engagement is to let individuals talk about their lived experiences of diseases and/or let representatives of advocacy and support organisations explain their ideas about developing an effective health programme. This also means to involve and approach community experts rather than relying exclusively on academic subject matter experts, which is traditionally still the norm. A good example of this is The Optimising Health Literacy (Ophelia) process, an intervention across eight health and community care organisations in Victoria, Australia using a collaborative or co-creative process of intervention identification and development (Batterham et al., 2014).

This, in turn, will have consequences in the ensuing planning stage for choice selection and strategy setting. Whereas in a traditional (often marketing-oriented) approach, conventional data collection designs (survey, focus group, randomised control trial) are used or intuitively the same orthodox processes and options are picked, changing to an equity-centred approach makes these choices questionable in terms of truly solving the problem, let alone for the community most affected. The Fighting Fit, Fighting Fat campaign in the UK comes to mind as an example where the traditional approach reached a traditional audience (those who already exercised and ate well) but not the priority group that the campaign aimed at. Besides reaching the "wrong" target, the traditional intervention might also miss the proverbial forest for the trees. Two examples from my local area may illustrate this.

An HIV-testing campaign directed at gay men and other men who have sex with men that specifically suggested a stress-free test centre experience did at first not see as many men use this service as expected. After debating attitudinal or behavioural obstinance or fear of exposure a round of community engagements brought to the fore a simple reason. Since these centres were only open during working hours and most members of this target segment work fulltime, they just could not get tested when the centre was open. The simple solution was to rearrange opening hours and include after-work, weekends, and lunch break times as well as vary location for easier commute. Now, clearly the other reasons were not irrelevant and still needed to be addressed and communicated properly, but it shows that getting hung up in a traditional cause-effect exercise to explain behaviour outcome with attitudinal, norm compliance, severity beliefs, or self-efficacy, a simpler reason for lack of the behaviour was overlooked.

The second example is not from our own area of health but the related social issues area of environmental protection. In general, the campaign had been determined to be a success. The New South Wales 'Hey Tosser' intervention is a state-wide anti-littering campaign by the state's Environment Protection Authority consisting of a multi-channel promotions campaign, an enforcement campaign allowing people to report littering when they see it, and partner activities with other government arms and the private sector. As I said, the campaign has been called effective on the usual measures (especially reporting littering and information search behaviour). Yet, a subsequent engagement with public transport commuters revealed that the absence of receptacles in public places (e.g., train platforms, bus stations, curb sides) was a chief reason for just leaving one's rubbish behind during commutes and work breaks. Now, this again neither invalidates all the other findings nor excuses an undesirable behaviour pattern, but it once again shows the oversight of a reasonably easy solution to adjust a target segment behaviour because of preconceived assumptions or biases and the lack of certain data collection engagements for planning purposes.

Generally, over the course of the previous chapter we have uncovered multiple general and group-specific traits that we need to become aware of and knowledgeable about to start planning communication campaigns both in terms of message content (the so-called creative execution) as well as message placement (the media and non-media selection for distribution of the message or messages). Next to the cognitive/rational factors that most behaviourist theories provide as well, one wants to collect some information on subconscious, values-based, experience-based, and affective or mood-related variables. Those factors combined have an impact on message decoding, i.e., how I read, comprehend, and relate to a message. And they also influence the probability, quality, and quantity of feedback the targeted receivers provide. This is expressed, of course, in 'proper' behaviour response, but also in the written and oral comments anyone makes about this intervention effort and its suggested behaviour.

In addition, a useful segmentation of message receivers is from human psychology theory, namely the need state level a person or group is at. There ought to be a big difference in our creative execution and appeal between trying to reach people in a safety level mindset and self-actualisation mindset. While the former would appreciate arguments that explain and assist with removal of dangers, the latter group would respond better to arguments that discuss achievements of individual esteem or potential. This does not only define and explain the receiver but probably illustrates the connection a group targeted in this manner has to the sender, the effect of channel noise, and the decoding process.

Drawing from multiple disciplines to redefine human health problems along a more humanistic or culture-inclusive understanding of human motivation is what I once described as a humanistic model of health communication (Werder, 2018). Such an approach adds actively listening, openness to other ideas and solicitation of input to the data collection and strategy preparation efforts in an inclusive manner. In turn, it offers deeper insights into the reasons for people's behaviours. This alone already provides additional information that is extremely useable in centrally produced health communication campaigns. However, the second crucial element is the ability to use those insights in helping people gain more self-awareness and formulate compelling arguments to consider for future behaviours. Help for self-help is a crucial element in a compassionate or egalitarian idea of resolving any personal or community concerns while growing and feeling good about being part of a group/community effort.

Nota Bene

This is certainly not the first and most likely not the last health communication title that suggest a more culturally appropriate and equitable effort when designing a health behaviour intervention. And there are signs around the world that some health promotion entities, including government types, have paid attention, and created campaigns that really aim to talk to a specific target audience in their 'language' and with their cultural practices and beliefs in mind.

But for the most part many health communication activities still maintain a top-down, factual evidence-based, risk-warning, and generalised format. This by itself underutilises the breadth and richness of language, human interaction, and even persuasive cues. But as I had mentioned in earlier chapters, even if a communication activity addressed at individual behaviour modification is done decently well, it by itself cannot offset decades of neglect and underinvestment in the healthcare sector in terms of access, training, and prevention support (e.g., safe environments) to the most vulnerable and voiceless. It is why efforts such as Health in All Policies are so appealing to me as a communicator.

Second, even if one were to tell a story rather than provide a list of data points, it is equally important to get away from an overuse of listing risk factors and negative consequences. While this is how the nightly news show functions (only a dramatic story is a good story), it is not how commercial adverting functions—and it is the latter that was the model for social marketing tactics. Brand advertising aims to provide as many positive factors as it can squeeze in the thirty seconds of a typical commercial to make the brand appealing. Our equivalent would be a listing of protective factors or positive consequences of the healthy behaviour.

Although the social marketing approach has become attractive to health communicators the moment it became ubiquitously known, it often is not practised to its utmost potential. While I do not believe it is useful to always go back to in all instances, even social marketing approaches are restricted by the nature of the workplace reality of its users. Practitioners in public health communication are, after all, public servants, or, if working for an NGO or related entity, funded by public institutions. As such, they must work with limited budgets and other resources and achieve their goal in a comparably short timeframe. It leads many to default to methods that have somewhat worked in the past.

But creativity in strategic communication is not about large budgets nor an army of people working for a long time to set something up. It is about idea generation (maybe in a criticism-free brainstorming sessions?); connection with one's intended audience on a deeper level so any advice sounds more trustworthy; modification of message tone aligned with foreseeable emotional state of the respective audience; and, finally, use of clear and familiar language, which not only assists in reducing the health literacy barrier but also makes a message more inclusive. The last two points include the connection of health and stigma. Communicate Health (2023) summarised fittingly how one wants to take this phenomenon into consideration when creating intervention campaigns:

> *Our health is extremely personal, and for some of us—whether it's because of our gender identity, sexual orientation, ability, race and ethnicity, health status, economic status, or other lived experience—it can be a source of shame. As health communicators, we know that stigma and shame get in the way of good health decisions and make it harder for people to access and understand health information. So counter stigma and shame in your writing by* ***normalizing a diverse range of human experiences and acknowledging barriers to health behaviors.*** (My highlights).

A culture-inclusive communication, therefore, should look towards health and medical humanities frameworks to seed the specific intervention. It ought to be clear about people's social routine practices to create interventions that reflect lived experiences and honed assessment. And finally, it should consider using culturally embedded narratives for promotional effort as those would not only be more engaging, likeable, and appealing, but would also transport receives into identification with the narrative characters or story which impacts behaviour change positively. If I can identify with what a character goes through to overcome an illness or prevent one by struggling to change a habit, I am more readily inclined to act on such a message. Moreover, it has a larger potential to achieve a grassroots-level social proliferation of the suggested behaviour (Larkey & Hecht, 2010), i.e., people start talking about it with their friends and relatives—and there is nothing more powerful than word-of-mouth promotion.

Ultimately, this does include assessing who is involved in the health communication activities. At best, the agency employs a diverse workforce, including those in leadership positions. If engaged with a particular community, whether it is ethnic or lifestyle, or ability-based, consider how hiring people from those communities benefits the efforts. There is an advantage in having people who 'look and sound' like the communities one serves to do the communicating. If this is not possible, maybe an external subcontracted agency, working primarily with certain communities and usually staffed by individuals from that group, can be employed. At a minimum, use community partners as consultants to identify priorities and acceptance prior to the development and distribution of the communicative output.

In general, the discussion of culture and cultural competency in programme design and execution is a fitting topic to highlight the breadth of communication that to date is mostly restricted to strategic or promotional (and often mediated) communication. Although interpersonal communication is making some inroads in the patient-facing communication training of young doctors, other communicative areas, such as organisational communication, nonverbal communication, intercultural communication, rhetorical criticism, media literacy, applied communication, performance studies, and visual communication tend to play a negligible role in health communication literature, let alone practice.

The issue of differences in fundamental concepts of health and comprehension of health information across various cultures and subcultures is an indicator that a broader usage of communication knowledge deserves further attention for health programme design and implementation.

We ought not forget that health promotion, especially in the arena of NCDs (non-communicable diseases) focuses upon encouraging the public to exercise behaviours which help develop and maintain their personal health. In that context, cultural dynamics play a central role for communicative interventions. As I discussed in Chap. 3 and will further explore in the next chapter, self-identity, group values, social norms, routine practices, body image, and the like influence particular health behaviours. They also vary across (sub-)cultures as their own creation are the consequence of the environments in which people grow up, live, and work. Given their social learning background suggests a broader application of sociological theories and approaches beyond Bandura's social learning model rather than a strict focus on cognitive-behavioural psychology theories.

Abel (2007) also rightfully points out that health promotion "*appears to be torn between its new health centred paradigm on the one side and primarily illness or risk centred empirical data on the other*" (p. 44). Although, as I outlined in Chap. 5, health promotion has begun highlighting the issue of well-being since the 1986 WHO meeting, the data it uses are still very much representative of disease-based epidemiological models. When the discussion turns to inequality, it essentially means inequality in illness, not inequality in the ability to stay healthy. For health communication output to advance the second idea requires from public health research, policy, and promotion to refocus on "*the distribution of health rather than disease and to include theories [and strategies] explanations on social inequalities in the means for producing health at the societal and the individual level*" (Abel, 2007, p. 44).

Next to the top-down, one-size-fits-all communication thinking, the disease focus is the other major hurdle for reaching individuals and communities of interest. It is where a different understanding of communication—from information dissemination and education/persuasion to idea sharing and joint solution generation—can make the greatest impact.

References

Abel, T. (2007). Cultural capital in health promotion. In D. McQueen, I. Kickbusch, L. Potvin, J. Pelikan, L. Balbo, & T. Abel (Eds.), *Health and modernity: The role of theory in health promotion* (pp. 43–73). Springer. https://doi.org/10.1007/978-0-387-37759-9_5

Al-Bannay, H., Jarus, T., Jongbloed, L., Yazigi, M., & Dean, E. (2014). Culture as a variable in health research: Perspectives and caveats. *Health Promotion International, 29*(3), 549–557. https://doi.org/10.1093/heapro/dat002

Attum, B., Hafiz, S., Malik, A., & Shamoon, Z. (2023, Updated July 3). Cultural competence in the care of Muslim patients and their families. In: *StatPearls [internet]*. Treasure Island (FL): StatPearls publishing. https://www.ncbi.nlm.nih.gov/books/NBK499933

Ayre, J., Muscat, D., Mac, O., Bonner, C., Dunn, A., Dalmazzo, J., Mouwad, D., & McCaffery, K. (2023). Helping patient educators meet health literacy needs: End-user testing and iterative development of an innovative health literacy editing tool. *PEC Innovation, 2*, 100162. https://doi.org/10.1016/j.pecinn.2023.100162

Batterham, R., Buchbinder, R., Beauchamp, A., Dodson, S., Elsworth, G., & Osborne, R. (2014). The OPtimising HEalth LIterAcy (Ophelia) process: Study protocol for using health literacy profiling and community engagement to create and implement health reform. *BMC Public Health, 14*(1) https://link.gale.com/apps/doc/A539593321/AONE?u=usyd&sid=bookmark-AONE&xid=a73c57ce

Bond, C., Mukandi, B., & Kajlich, H. (2021). *Social and cultural determinants of health. Renewing Queensland's alcohol and other drugs plan – Consultation paper*. Queensland Mental Health Commission.

Braveman, P., Arkin, E., Orleans, T., Proctor, D., & Plough, A. (2017). *What is health equity? And what difference does a definition make?* Robert Wood Johnson Foundation.

Campbell, C., & Murray, M. (2004). Community health psychology: Promoting analysis and action for social change. *Journal of Health Psychology, 9*(2), 187–195.

CommunicateHealth. (2023, March 9). A framework for equity-centered health communication. CommunicateHealth. https://communicatehealth.com/wp-content/uploads/ch-echc-framework.pdf

Duncan, E. (2017, December 21). *Culture-centered approach for community-driven health communication – An interview with professor Mohan Jyoti Dutta.* Frontiers-Science News. https://blog.frontiersin.org/2017/12/21/mohan-jyoti-dutta-culture-centered-community-driven-health-communication/

Dutta, M. (2007). *Communicating health: A culture-centered approach.* Polity Press.

Ford, J., Grasso, D., Elhai, J., & Courtois, C. (2015). Social, cultural, and other diversity issues in the traumatic stress field. In *Posttraumatic stress disorder* (2nd ed., pp. 503–546). Academic. https://doi.org/10.1016/B978-0-12-801288-8.00011-X

Fremeaux, I. (2005). New labour's appropriation of the concept of community: A critique. *Community Development Journal, 40*(3), 265–274.

Fulk, J., Steinfield, C., Schmitz, J., & Power, J. (1987). A social information processing model of media use in organizations. *Communication Research, 14*(5), 529–552. https://doi.org/10.1177/009365087014005005

George, E., Mackean, T., Baum, F., & Fisher, M. (2019). Social determinants of indigenous health and indigenous rights in policy: A scoping review and analysis of problem representation. *International Indigenous Policy Journal, 10*(2) https://doi.org/10.18584/iipj.2019.10.2.4

Gutchess, A., & Rajaram, S. (2023). Consideration of culture in cognition: How we can enrich methodology and theory. *Psychonomic Bulletin & Review, 30*(3), 914–931. https://doi.org/10.3758/s13423-022-02227-5

Guttman, N., & Salmon, C. (2004). Guilt, fear, stigma and knowledge gaps: Ethical issues in public health communication interventions. *Bioethics, 18*(6), 531–552. https://doi.org/10.1111/j.1467-8519.2004.00415.x

Hall, S. (1980). Encoding/decoding. In Centre for Contemporary Cultural Studies (Ed.), *Culture, media, language: Working papers in cultural studies, 1972–79* (pp. 128–138). Hutchinson.

Hall, S. (1997). *Representation: Cultural representations and signifying practices*. Sage.

Hofstede, G. (1980). *Culture's consequences: International differences in work-related values*. Sage.

Howarth, C. (2011). Representations, identity and resistance in communication. In D. Hook, B. Franks, & M. Bauer (Eds.), *The social psychology of communication* (pp. 153–158). Palgrave Macmillan.

Hsieh, E., & Kramer, E. (2021). *Rethinking culture in health communication*. Wiley-Blackwell.

Iwelunmor, J., & Airhihenbuwa, C. (2017, January 25). Culture, a social determinant of health and risk: Considerations for health and risk messaging. *Oxford research encyclopedia of communication*. https://oxfordre.com/communication/view/10.1093/acrefore/9780190228613.001.0001/acrefore-9780190228613-e-221

Kostygina, G., Tran, H., Binns, S., Szczypka, G., Emery, S., Vallone, D., & Hair, E. (2020). Boosting health campaign reach and engagement through use of social media influencers and memes. *Social Media + Society, 6*(2). https://doi.org/10.1177/2056305120912475

Kripalani, S., Jacobson, T., Mugalla, I., Cawthon, C., Niesner, K., & Vaccarino, V. (2010). Health literacy and the quality of physician-patient communication during hospitalization. *Journal of Hospital Medicine, 5*(5), 269–275. https://doi.org/10.1002/jhm.667

Larkey, L., & Hecht, M. (2010). A model of effects of narrative as culture-centric health promotion. *Journal of Health Communication, 15*(2), 114–135. https://doi.org/10.1080/10810730903528017

Lewis, B., & Lewis, J. (2015). *Health communication: A media and cultural studies approach*. Palgrave.

Liburd, L., Namageyo-Funa, A., & Jack, L., Jr. (2007). Understanding "masculinity" and the challenges of managing type-2 diabetes among African American men. *Journal of the National Medical Association, 99*(5), 550–558.

Manderson, L., & Allotey, P. (2003). Storytelling, marginality, and community in Australia: How immigrant position their difference in health care settings. *Medical Anthropology, 22*, 1–21. https://doi.org/10.1080/014597403901782371

Moscovici, S. (1961/2008). Psychoanalysis: Its image and its public. Polity Press. (First published as La psychanalyse, son image et son public. Paris: Presses universitaires de France.)

Mutair, A., Plummer, V., O'Brien, A., & Clerehan, R. (2014). Providing culturally congruent care for Saudi patients and their families. *Contemporary Nurse, 46*(2), 254–258. https://doi.org/10.5172/conu.2014.46.2.254

Osborn, C., Paasche-Orlow, M., Bailey, S., & Wolf, M. (2011). The mechanisms linking health literacy to behavior and health status. *American Journal of Health Behavior, 35*(1), 118–128. https://doi.org/10.5993/ajhb.35.1.11

Porter, R., & Samovar, L. (Eds.). (1988). *Intercultural communication: A reader* (5th ed.). Wadsworth Publishing Company.

Rateau, P., Tavani, J., & Delouvèe, S. (2023). Social representations of the coronavirus and causal perception of its origin: The role of reasons for fear. *Health: An Interdisciplinary Journal for the Social Study of Health, Illness and Medicine, 27*(1), 94–113. https://doi.org/10.1177/13634593211005172

Russell, K. (2015, February 13). 'Left swipe Dat' music video uses tinder to raise tobacco awareness. *USA Today Newspaper* (College blog section). https://www.usatoday.com/story/college/2015/02/13/left-swipe-dat-music-video-uses-tinder-to-raise-tobacco-awareness/37400689/

Saitz, R. (2018). Community-based participatory research: Advocacy or approach? *American Journal of Public Health, 108*(12), 1578–1579. https://doi.org/10.2105/AJPH.2018.304739

Salmon, C., Wooten, K., Gentry, E., Cole, G., & Kroger, F. (1996). AIDS knowledge gaps in the first decade of the epidemic. *Journal of Health Communication, 1*(2), 141–155. https://doi.org/10.1080/108107396128112

Shoemaker, S., Wolf, M., & Brach, C. (2014). Development of the patient education materials assessment tool (PEMAT): A new measure of understandability and actionability for print and audiovisual patient information. *Patient Education and Counseling, 96*(3), 395–403. https://doi.org/10.1016/j.pec.2014.05.027

Smith, P., & Bond, M. (2022). Four decades of challenges by culture to mainstream psychology: Finding ways forward. *Journal of Cross-Cultural Psychology, 53*(7–8), 729–751. https://doi.org/10.1177/00220221221084041

Sørensen, K., Van den Broucke, S., Fullam, J., Doyle, G., Pelikan, J., Slonska, Z., Brand, H., & (HLS-EU) Consortium Health Literacy Project European. (2012). Health literacy and public health: A systematic review and integration of definitions and models. *BMC Public Health, 12*, 80. https://doi.org/10.1186/1471-2458-12-80

Stephens, C. (2007). Community as practice: Social representations of community and their implications for health promotion. *Journal of Community & Applied Social Psychology, 17*(2), 103–114. https://doi.org/10.1002/casp.884

Sussman, A., Montoya, C., Werder, O., Davis, S., Wallerstein, N., & Kong, A. (2013). An adaptive CBPR approach to create weight management materials for a school-based health center intervention. *Journal of Obesity, 2013*, 978482. https://doi.org/10.1155/2013/978482

Truth Initiative. (2015). *Inspiring tobacco-free lives – Annual Report.* Truth Initiative.

Vaughn, E., & Krenz, V. (2013). Planning, implementing, and evaluating culturally appropriate programs. In M. Pèrez & R. Luquis (Eds.), *Public health/AAHE: Cultural competence in health education and health promotion* (2nd ed., pp. 171–180). Jossey-Bass.

Viswanath, K., Finnegan, J., Hannan, P., & Luepker, R. (1991). Health and knowledge gaps: Some lessons from the Minnesota heart health program. *American Behavioral Scientist, 34*(6), 712–726. https://doi.org/10.1177/0002764291034006008

Wallerstein, N., Duran, B., Oetzel, J., & Minkler, M. (2018). *Community-based participatory research for health: Advancing social and health equity* (3rd ed.). Jossey-Bass.

Werder, O. (2018). Toward a humanistic model in health communication. *Global Health Promotion, 26*(1), 33–40. https://doi.org/10.1177/1757975916683385

Williams, D. (2003). The health of men: Structured inequalities and opportunities. *American Journal of Public Health, 93*(5), 724–731. https://doi.org/10.2105/AJPH.93.5.724

World Health Organisation. (2022). *Health literacy development for the prevention and control of noncommunicable diseases: Volume 1. Overview.* WHO.

World Health Organization. (2008). *Closing the gap in a generation: Health equity through action on the social determinants of health: Final report of the commission on social determinants of health.* WHO. https://www.who.int/publications/i/item/WHO-IER-CSDH-08.1

World Health Organization. (2020, December 24). *10 global health issues to track in 2021.* Spotlight News Report. WHO. https://www.who.int/news-room/spotlight/10-global-health-issues-to-track-in-2021

Zoller, H., & Dutta, M. (2008). *Emerging perspectives in health communication: Meaning, culture, and power.* Routledge.

Part III

Transformative Thinking in Communicating Health

7

Nurturing a Shared Vision: Self-identity, Relationship Building, and People-Powered Interventions

Overview

Some years ago, when I was working in advertising in the United States, I had become curious about how any of the local megachurches pull so many people each week to their services after reading an article about the megachurch phenomenon in the local newspaper. Since I didn't live too far away from one of them at the time, I decided to attend one of their services in their cavernous, almost stadium-like building. Although I do not call myself overly religious, I had grown up in my local church and was familiar with the idea of a church community and what motivator this is for many to stay connected. After that service—although conducted in a modern, some might say engrossing, others might say spectacular fashion—it left me wondering how this mass of people (I guessed between 3000 and 5000) would be a true community since they seemed to have come from all over the city and dispersed afterwards.

Years later I came across Duhigg's (2012) book, *The Power of Habit*, and while reading the chapter on habits of societies, where he used the Saddleback megachurch in California, founded by Rick Warren, next to

O. Werder, *Transformational Health Communication*,
https://doi.org/10.1007/978-981-99-9606-3_7

the Civil Rights movement in the United States as an example, I remembered my own experience and questions. In his chapter, Duhigg shed some light on why those two groups as well as probably the church I had frequented succeed. There are two key aspects, which—I would argue—could equally work for health-related behaviours (or shall I call it healthy habits?).

One, achieving not only a new behaviour but a sustainable one requires leveraging the power of social habits, i.e., getting people to take responsibility for their new habit. It is something I discussed more extensively in Chap. 3. And two, to make those new behaviours self-perpetuating, it requires to (a) make them an aspect of people's social experience and daily lives and (b) figure out a way to teach people how they then can work out where to go on their own. For Saddleback Church, this was small (neighbourhood) groups for weekday bible study as well as curricula and workshops where small groups members learn how to run a faith-based meeting circle without being guided by a pastor or priest (Duhigg, 2012, p. 239).

Like the events following the Montgomery bus boycott and the work of Martin Luther King, the conversion of people from followers into self-directed leaders in the megachurch has created a movement through which people felt a new sense of identity. Ever since I started thinking about how to improve or transform health communication, I recalled these examples and started wondering how to recreate these sequences for health behaviours. For instance, in any gym I ever was a member of I always noticed the clear difference between those people who could easily stop at any moment and those for who the gym (or exercise in it) has become a way of life. While the former group would absolutely need to have some ongoing guidance and motivator, like a personal trainer, to stay active, the latter tend to work through their rigorous weight or other programme religiously on their own. Those two segments do not really differ in demographics, psychographics, or lifestyle in general. It is just that one group has made gym exercise part of their identity and the other has not. This begs the question, what is self-identity and how do we make a health habit part of someone's identity?

Self-identity and Behaviour

As the literature into the sequential relationship between identity formation and behaviour shows, there is benefit in understanding how human identity is formulated and reformulated (Côtè, 1996). By and large, identity is defined as an enduring and salient part of one's internalised perception of self (Rise et al., 2010). It assists with overcoming chaos by determining how we think and feel about ourselves and as such conveys specific meaning(s) and stability to one's behaviour (Graybiel, 2008; Obschonka et al., 2015). It is in fact a major source of stability of behaviour and is regarded as the precedent to behaviour. An example is thinking about oneself in a way related to action (e.g., I am an athlete, so I work out) (Savickas, 2002). Yet, a person's self-concept comprises different role identities (e.g., employee, partner, and spouse) (Stryker & Burke, 2000), some of which are self-defined and -nurtured (such as the 'I am an athlete' self-identity schema), others are derived from belonging to—or wanting to belong to—a social group or organisation. Subsequently, identity encompasses expectations of one's social position. This is known as the role-person merger, the degree to which one identifies as something (person, group of people, community, or organisation). The extent to which a societal role is internalised within a person determines the balance between "Me" and "We" information, whereby the latter denotes how someone derives her own identity from identifying with something such as a person, group of people, community, or organisation (Simons, 2021; Thoits & Virshup, 1997).

This in turn connects and contrasts different purposes of a role. While one might adopt a self-image that best leads to a personal goal or desire, it also serves to regulate how one ought to act in a situation. This latter part has been called the logic of appropriateness by March (1994), by which "*a decision maker considers what rules specify what a person with a particular identity does in a particular situation.*" It, in short, becomes a means of social adaptation to each other in a group situation. In either case, the objective is to find a meaningful interpretation of a fundamentally ambiguous environment.

Research efforts in social identity and social psychology (Melucci, 1995; Polletta & Jasper, 2001) have shown the interplay between individual identity and habit-forming through external social environments. There are also arguments that if a behaviour has been performed repeatedly in the past and is thus under habitual control, then decisions to engage in it in the future depend more on the importance of the behaviour for the person's self-identity than on judgements and feelings about the behaviour (e.g., attitudes) or the perceived expectations of others (the so-called subjective norms) (Charng et al., 1988; Terry et al., 1999). While some of the often-cited cognitive-behaviourist theories used as platforms for health communication campaigns pick up on some of the interdependent identity assessments—the Theory of Reasoned Action (Ajzen & Fishbein, 1973) introduced the subjective norms expectation variable and the Social Cognitive Theory (Bandura, 1986), the interplay of outcome expectations and norms and influences of others variables—the independent self-identity concept and its determining force in health(!) behaviour formation have been explored by only a few studies (Michie et al., 2011; Verplanken & Faes, 1999; West, 2007).

To pick up on an earlier example about individuals changing to engaging in more regular physical activity, once exercise becomes an aspect of people's identity and they start to define themselves as a gym rat, runner, or swimmer (an element of identity known as a label or attribute), they do not only exercise on a regular basis but sustain this behaviour without being prompted. This follows the Applied Social Identity Approach (ASIA; Haslam, 2014), which calls for understanding how social identities are related to individuals' attitudes and behaviours. Comparatively, studies in political communication have shown that political messages usually only affect people when those people possess the same identities of those who have created the messages while attempts to influence others have often been futile (Tarrant et al., 2012). Yet this finding is not exclusive to the political arena. Campaigns asking for preventative action (e.g., getting the annual flu shot) resonate more with those for who annual health check-ups and a desire to catch any health irregularity early are part of their health or self-preservation identity. Finally, the concept of collective identity is not-surprisingly also a hallmark of new social movements (Melucci, 1996) as people who join such a movement have adopted an ideology and constructed an identity that in their view justifies their actions.

Insights from New Social Movement Theory

Starting in the 1960s new social movements (NSMs) appeared that were seen as "new" in contrast to the "old" working-class movement. Whereas the latter are identified by Marxist theory as the major challenger to capitalist society, the new social movements are organised around gender, race, ethnicity, youth, sexuality, spirituality, countercultures, environmentalism, animal rights, pacifism, human rights, and the like. In the 1980s, new social movement theory (NSMT) emerged in Europe to analyse this phenomenon (Buechler, 2013).

The centrality of collective identity in those new social remonstrations (Johnston et al., 1994) make it worthwhile to examine public resistance movements. That is, new social movements draw their ability to engage in collective action from their ability to construct a collective social identity in the first place (Melucci, 1989), focusing on their respective issues related to everyday life, civil society, and the cultivation of "free spaces" (Buechler, 2013). Without going too deep into the rabbit hole of critical social movement philosophy, it is noteworthy that these new social movements have been explained as "*being concerned with quality of life, self-realization, identity formation, moral autonomy and political participation*" (Habermas, 1987) and places for "*new collective identities connecting personal needs and movement participation*" to promote "*democratisation in society and in everyday life*" (Melucci, 1989).

It is comprehensible that some still wonder what all this has to do with public health, let alone health communication. I refer these sceptics to documented overt public opposition to health practices. For example, the 2014 Ebola crisis in Central and West Africa saw local resistance and public tension in impacted local villages and communities to state-organised public health efforts (Garrett, 2015) that have been explained as a response to "*cultural norms and narratives learned through long histories of state interventions that were far from beneficent*" (Bulled & Puffer, 2017).

Understanding the importance of public reactions to health programmes and efforts has first been recognised as an issue as early as the 1950s that eventually engendered the field of critical medical anthropology. One of the key ideas of the seminal work by Paul (1955) was that data and health information are the product of interpretations and cultural lenses applied by the receivers of the efforts. Since social relationships influence health as much as individual personality and ecological status, it is these (often unequal) social structures that we ought to pay more attention to.

Narrowing the general idea of new social movements, namely democratisation of society and participation, to public health, we arrive at the notion of the social origins of illness and unequal valued status and access to care. It is both issues of poverty, pollution, and violence as contributors to poor health as well as the origins of dominant cultural constructions of health (e.g., a preference for individual pay-for-care models reinforcing access inequalities in individualistic cultures) that potentially lead to push-back and resistance but also offer communicative avenues if properly understood. As Bulled and Puffer (2017) conclude, "*health is intertwined with the social, the political, the economic, the moral, and the historic*" (p. 4).

Communities protesting the intrusion of biomedically based public health efforts have in fact a long history. The suspicion of vaccines or compliant behaviour during an epidemic are examples that saw—and still see—not only passive resistance (by, e.g., not following health orders or getting vaccinated) but at times overt opposition. I recall street rallies in many countries during the COVID pandemic where people openly protested the lockdowns and social distancing orders by marching through the streets. They highlight the struggle between the common good and individual rights and the ongoing need for negotiation between the different interpretation of ideas, approaches, and medical advancements. The values-based inclusion of politics I discussed in an earlier chapter adds more complexity and often division that provide further bases for contest. To overcome at least some of these issues requires an understanding of health problems from the perspective of the people. In that sense, taking a cue from how to engage and negotiate with social movements provides a fitting analogy or training module for the task at hand.

Community Engagement Through Communication

Communication is a regular human activity since we as humans are drawn to one another and communicate with each other in a variety of capacities. At the same token, as I explained above, we fill several roles or identities over just the course of a single day and so our communication depends on the context of an interaction. The two key elements people perceive as producing an effective communicative interaction are the use of clear and understandable message delivery and an attempt to create and maintain lasting and genuine relationships through communication. While the former reduces or eliminates misunderstanding or alteration of messages, in turn decreasing possible conflict, the latter picks up if such dissonance happens after all by being a key factor in resolving misunderstanding and other natured conflict in a respectful manner. In short, communication is effective when it leaves everyone involved content and feeling accomplished.

Now, to feel accomplished in a communicative interaction requires that one participates in that interaction. This means for community-oriented (or target group-oriented) health messages that people of a group or community are somewhat involved in communication strategy and, in fact, encouraged to take ownership of initiatives of a development instead of thinking of themselves as recipients of a target behaviour call-to-action. Findings in studies related to risk and disaster relief communication show that good communication practices in community engagement involve *participation and feedback of community members* and *strengthening accountability to affected communities* (Le Bou et al., 2021).

These concepts are of central concern for a research area, known as participatory research, a research perspective that has social action and structural change as its ultimate goals. Whereas the most used term, community-based participatory research (CBPR), was advanced by public health, it traces its origins to community psychology, which has enjoyed a rich history of participatory, collaborative research efforts (Kral & Allen, 2016). In traditional public health research, including health promotion, community members have typically been the objects of research that generates representational knowledge, with the research problems studied being those identified by individuals from outside of the community. In participatory approaches, community members transform representational knowledge into relational and reflective knowledge through the establishment of a democratic dialogue with the researcher (Gustavsen et al., 2008; Kral & Allen, 2016). The benefit of such an approach stems from the simple principle that communities—no matter how defined—are composed of people who know each other, respect each other, and communicate with each other.

If an outsider—here a researcher—aims to obtain information from the community, they will inevitably discuss and evaluate the researcher and her requests, and collectively decide if they want to participate. More importantly, they ask how they and their community might benefit from such participation, a question that is particularly an issue with communities that are marginalised, have unequal power and access, or have experienced exploitation in some form or another. What participatory research offers is a perspective that acknowledges these realities and effectively uses them to reduce barriers of adoption and participation.

It is certainly true that most activities including community participation happen in academic research. Yet, the principles described are equally applicable and usable to and by professional practitioners in the health communication sector. As the reader may remember from our discussion in Chap. 5, the 1978 WHO Alma Ata conference laid the groundwork for legitimising the discussion of equitable '*social structures*' as a crucial antecedent to improving the health of human populations. In recent years, the initiation of the United Nations Sustainable Development Goals has further contributed to making community participation a priority in healthcare and prevention globally (Fox & Stoett, 2016). Although this has heightened the interest among healthcare and promotion practitioners to engage communities better, challenges remained.

As the substantial meta-analytical review by Haldane et al. (2019) has shown, "intra- and inter-organisational negotiating and learning, that over time results in 'trust' and 'authentic' relationships which ultimately drive partnerships forward"—called process outcomes in the study—are hugely relevant to create contextually appropriate interventions and ultimately improve the target community's health on an ongoing basis. It further emphasises the fact that community-participation interventions should not be misconstrued as a tool to improve health outcomes momentarily but should indeed be undertaken as a long-term and permanent process to implement and support health programmes to sustain these outcomes (Davison et al., 2013).

A successful application of this can be found in the Fiji COVID-19 emergency response project (2020) which from the outset included a stakeholder engagement plan (SEP). This plan included trust building between the public and Ministry of Health and Medical Services (MoHMS), proactive dissemination of risk information, transparency in communication, and active listening and engagement with the community (p. 8). As a result of executing the SEP along with other measures (lockdowns, border closure, curfews, tracing apps), Fiji remained largely COVID-free until April 2021 and only recorded cases from managed quarantine facilities. Human error in April 2021 despite everything led to some community outbreaks, but those were brought under control reasonably fast (Prakash, 2021). All in all, the early community involvement measures led to not only broad acceptance but active participation in keeping the country safe.

The net takeaway is that community engagement in health communication campaign design and execution not only offers a sense of responsibility by the targeted group towards resolving a crisis, risk, or condition but enhances self-reliance, critical reflection of information to make informed choices, and a more trusting relationship to health workers and government health education and promotion stakeholders.

Communicating a Shared Vision

What the above-mentioned topics translate to for health communication is a consideration of self-identity and self-actualisation drivers rather than a sole focus on attitudes and beliefs as explanatory factors for (un)healthy behaviour patterns. A model that may be helpful for this is the Communication Theory of Identity (CTI) (Hecht et al., 2004), which regards communication as an element rather than just a product of identity. It means that a person's sense of self is part of his or her social behaviour and the sense of self emerges and is defined and redefined in social interaction. CTI accordingly centres identity as relational and takes into consideration identity as a discursive process.

As my earlier discussions about the relationship between ideology, identity, framing, and collective behaviour as well as the work by Hecht and colleagues (Hecht, 2009; Hecht et al., 2004; Jung & Hecht, 2004) have shown, there is a connection between how human identity is formulated and reformulated and the creation of collective identities through discourse and dialogue. This connection has been seen equally as the reason for people resisting and rejecting attempts to sway health behaviour, and for a larger mobilisation and ongoing participation for many social issues, including public health.

While many health issues do not typically lead to political public action, the principles with which people participate in health movements and calls-to-action are similar, as public mobilisations in the past 2–3 years towards the health effects of environmental degradation and protest rallies for healthcare reforms have demonstrated. It is here where studies of new social movements contribute to the alignment of individual identity formation with group ideology, which then explain the behavioural action (here joining the movement and trying to influence others in turn).

What this all points to for our area is exploring the feasibility of individual-, small group-, or community-involved health communication as an opposite to centrally organised health communication, typically using a mediated message delivery format. Whereas the current utilised methods of interactive digital technology media use (to enable access to information and services) and media advocacy (a combination of mass media with community organising) suggest a more participatory approach, health communicators using them often struggle to understand the audiences they seek to reach and subsequently match messages and channels to observable social and behavioural characteristics (Freimuth & Quinn, 2004).

A deeper understanding of what determines and drives both individuals' and communities'(health) identities, in short, a more resolute inclusion of areas such as intercultural health communication, health-focused linguistics, and health sociology, has the distinct potential to close gaps. General work on the relationship between language use and identity have already demonstrated that identity plays a sizeable role in the way people express themselves in conversations, the symbols, and labels they use to talk about something, and the modes considered appropriate to talk about a topic (Llamas & Watt, 2010).

We know, for instance, that identity is neither a static nor a singular concept. As Hecht (2009) argued: "*One implication is that at any time we are likely to be experiencing multiple, intersecting identities, some of which are group-based or communal. People rarely operate out of a single identity; rather multiple identities guide their thoughts and behaviours*" (p. 140). Connected with that 'layered' perspective of how our identity is formed and why it remains acquiescent is the sense that communication is among the explanatory element in that process. As I had raised elsewhere, we need to transcend the notion that health communication is merely a strategy to reach a defined static target community. It is rather an ongoing contributor to a person's or group's identity formation in a specific setting. In turn, this identity is subsequently enacted through communication making the association reciprocal.

In that sense, it is "*critical to broaden the interdisciplinary nature of communication scholarship that examines individual and collective sense-making and action, and collective action and mobilisation driven by social actors embedded in institutional settings*" (Obregón & Tufte, 2017). This also means that we need to 'unlearn' aspects of strategic health communication. Whereas the idea of communication as a relational and dynamic process may be well-known, the dominant models of strategic health communication (including the entirety of social marketing approaches) focus still mostly on individual-level processes of change. Yet, the history and evolution of the HIV/AIDS movement, for instance, and how it impacted policy debates is an example of collective or group-driven communication processes and tactics (Stackpool-Moore, 2006).

Being a teacher, I have a perennial interest in figuring out what good teaching looks like. When I came across it many decades ago, I felt very strongly about the argumentation of Brazilian educator and philosopher Paulo Freire, who argued in his seminal work, Pedagogy of the Oppressed, that education is a "*means to building a 'critical consciousness' that would enable people to create change in their lives*" (Freire, 1970). I have aimed to model my teaching along these ideas because what Freire essentially argues is that a true educator needs to realise that meaning making requires open and equal communication, which moves the student from a passive receiver of information to an active partner in learning. Ultimately, the teacher becomes a guide in a self-learning and self-awareness growth experience the student goes through, whereby she not only reproduces the learnt material but creates her own understanding of it, including what it means in context, and what position towards a topic she holds and why.

I cannot help but see similarities in this to the current dominant health (and, for that matter, all social issues) communication approaches and how they could be transformed. Like the passive student, most people are aware of their health (behaviour) situation but don't make any effort to change it to the point that consider their situation something normal. Subsequently, top-down broad information dissemination or nudging appeals for change are noticed and possibly believed but not acted upon. On the contrary, a person who is encouraged to think, reflect, and contribute is creating her identity from the inside-out in connection with the social communities she interacts and belongs to. To arrive at that, a health communicator needs to establish dialogue with the targeted group. Since building rapport requires using the language with which the individuals of that group are familiar, it is necessary to integrate oneself into the life of the average individual, studying and employing their language, their practices, their beliefs, and their communication patterns and flow.

The conversion of Freire's thoughts on education to health communication is not revolutionary nor new as many scholars in our discipline have written about their usefulness to health behaviour influence over the years (Obregon & Mosquera, 2005; Schiavo, 2016; Wallerstein &

Bernstein, 1988; Wiggins, 2012), addressing health equity, empowerment via participatory approaches, community engagement during crises and risks, health literacy, interactive media use, and capacity building and training to improve patient-provider communication. Yet, especially in the so-called industrialised world, their potential remains unrealised in mainstream public health circles.

Hence, participatory and identity-oriented approaches seem to provide an improvement for health intervention efforts. There are numerous examples that inside-out, group-, and self-identity adjusted behaviour interventions have not only better recall and uptake but longer sustainability among the targeted community. This can be traced back to the interaction of self-image, self-awareness, and self-esteem with three important interpersonal needs I touched upon when talking about human psychology, human motivation, and Maslow's (1943) hierarchy of needs. The need for control/respect, the need for inclusion/belonging, and the need for affection affect how we communicate with other people.

In addressing and meeting those needs, the targeted community begins assisting the health communicator with creating an effective programme directed at them. To engage a community in that manner does not require from the health communicator to relearn everything and abandon all learnt promotion principles, tactical media, and non-media operations or whatever else one does. But it does mean that the health communicator moves from a teacher or expert of health education and behaviour risks to a collaborator or guide in grasping best practices and communication choices along with the targeted group members. This attitudinal shift would make communication not just more inclusive but most likely more rewarding for everyone because it not only provides a framework for health message creation but also helps in better understanding people's health practices.

Final Thoughts

Growing up in Germany, I remember my grandfather always saying, "*Der Ton macht die Musik*" (literal translation: 'the sound makes the music') when someone threw dozens of arguments at him in an ever-increasing frenzied pitch to adopt that person's opinion. What he was getting at, of course, is how this saying also figuratively translates into English, namely '*It's not what you say, but how you say it.*'

Since many non-communicable disease campaigns aim to prevent future diseases by promoting healthy habits or lifestyles—for instance smoking, food, weight control, alcohol abuse, other drug consumption—they face the immense twin barrier of (a) having to address people who due to good health at the time are little motivated to listen and (b) the fact that the enactment of the suggested behaviour (or their avoidance) may have little to do with concepts of health. People, for instance, exercise for other reasons (especially if it pertains to competitive team sports), they may have moral positions towards alcohol and drugs, and so on. As Blaxter (2010) concluded, "*the basic lessons of health promotion [are universally] accepted, and those who behave 'unhealthily' are as likely—if not more likely—to be aware of dangers*" (p. 90). People may find excuses, but they are not ignorant of the effects of their actions. So, there appears to be some need to not only find the right argument but also the right tone to break through.

It is for that reason that I have asked to reflect more deeply on what address format appeals to what person or group. This differs greatly between people based on their self-perception and role definition whereby some accept and even prefer to be a passive recipient of a behavioural appeal and others to be an active agent in a discourse scenario. It brings to the fore the importance of self-identity as one critical aspect of how one wishes to being communicated to. This is far from borrowing gimmicky tricks from commercial persuasion such as humour or fast-paced action in a mediated behaviour change campaign.

It rather relates to something we called '*bridging the gap between the real and ideal self*' in my days in advertising whereby the advertised brand becomes the hero moving you to—or at least close to—the ideal self-image. If, say, you want to be more liked or loved, this fashion or fragrance brand can facilitate that. In the same vein, displaying a healthy behaviour to others in your in-group, or actively trying to convince a loved one that a behaviour change is beneficial caters to the 'better person,' 'caring relative or friend,' or even 'the cool person others want to be with' persona ideals.

This idea was applied, for example, in the *Truth* anti-tobacco campaign aimed at eliminating teen smoking and developed and steered by the Florida Tobacco Program from 1998 to 2003 and later adopted by the national Truth Initiative (formerly known as American Legacy Foundation). To counter the appeal of smoking on youths as a tool for rebellion and empowerment, the programme encouraged teens to rebel against the manipulation of tobacco companies. It did so by collaborating directly with Florida youths to co-develop this campaign as it was speaking to their own generation. One result of using this participatory approach that looked deeper into why teens smoke and/or ignore the traditional warnings was the campaign name itself. Teens described their ideal campaign as one that would tell them the truth about tobacco. Plus, it also worked very well. Multiple evaluative studies between 2000 and 2009 found declining smoker rates, declining intentions to smoke among non-smokers, and a positive correlation between campaign exposure and smoking uptake risk (Farrelly et al., 2002; Holtgrave et al., 2009; National Cancer Institute, 2008; Vallone et al., 2018).

The example is illustrative of both the *personal layer* and the *enacted layer* in Hecht et al.'s (2004) communication theory of identity framework. The former layer connects with the cognitive-behaviourist theories, I mentioned earlier in this chapter, and especially Bandura's concept of self-efficacy, or the belief that one can perform a learned behaviour (Bandura, 1977). This self-directed motivation regards behaviour adoption as an end goal or a means to an end to maintain good health. In the latter layer a health behaviour message serves to educate individuals about how to claim a desired identity by showcasing a certain identity through specific actions.

Moreover, there are two insights from studying social movements and the grassroots groups who create and run them. One, communication practices within communities draw on formal and informal communication networks as a space of learning and growth for activism and collective action. While most health topics are not heavily politically charged, we have seen cases where ordinary citizens who are affected in one way or another by a health crisis took communication into their own hands—often literally, using digital and mobile media—and rejected being passive "beneficiaries" of institutional health communication campaigns (Barbas & Postill, 2017). This title mentioned a few, such as protests to COVID safe behaviour requirements by governments and the ongoing debate around childhood (and other) vaccination.

Two, emerging work on communicating for participating in social change (Chattoo & Feldman, 2017) found that different types of narratives have the potential to trigger greater public engagement than factual evidence. Being absorbed in a narrative—known as transportation—reduces cognitive resistance to persuasive messages embedded within the narrative (Green & Brock, 2000) and accordingly has been linked to changes in audiences' knowledge, attitudes, and behaviour (Murphy et al., 2013). Subsequently storytelling, with a strong focus on human stories, can be an effective support tool in the search for public engagement and acquiescence. While not in the same arena as what team sports fans or political party activists experience, a captivating human story about saving or restoring health and overcoming illness still contributes quite well to identity formation and group belonging. Relating to and connecting with other people enhances the human desire to belong, which in turn boosts self-esteem, improves psychological and behavioural functioning, and improves the meaning of our lives. In short, it positively influences well-being.

The ideas and premises advanced in this chapter point to a need for a greater focus on interdisciplinary approaches and theoretic frameworks in the examination of communication phenomena and their connections to health attitudes and behaviours. For instance, we ought to follow with interest what findings emerge in the ongoing quest to understand how communication processes shape the formation and evolution of social movements and their contributions to change. To date, there is limited knowledge how deeply healthcare and promotions organisations and bodies understand and embrace the role of communication in their public health mission.

References

Ajzen, I., & Fishbein, M. (1973). Attitudinal and normative variables as predictors of specific behavior. *Journal of Personality and Social Psychology, 27*, 41–57.

Bandura, A. (1977). Self-efficacy: Toward a unifying theory of behavior change. *Psychological Review, 84*, 191–215.

Bandura, A. (1986). *Social foundations of thought and action: A social cognitive theory*. Prentice-Hall.

Barbas, A., & Postill, J. (2017). Communication activism as a school of politics: Lessons from Spain's indignados movement. *Journal of Communication, 67*(5), 646–664. https://doi.org/10.1111/jcom.12321

Blaxter, M. (2010). *Health* (2nd ed.). Polity Press.

Buechler, S. (2013). New social movements and new social movement theory. In D. Snow, D. Della Porta, B. Klandermans, & D. McAdam (Eds.), *The Wiley-Blackwell encyclopedia of social and political movements*. Wiley-Blackwell. https://doi.org/10.1002/9780470674871.wbespm143

Bulled, N., & Puffer, M. (2017). Introduction. In N. Bulled (Ed.), *Thinking through resistance: A study of public oppositions to contemporary global health practice* (pp. 1–21). Routledge.

Charng, H., Piliavin, J., & Callero, P. (1988). Role identity and reasoned action in the prediction of repeated behaviour. *Social Psychology Quarterly, 51*(4), 303–317. https://doi.org/10.2307/2786758

Chattoo, C., & Feldman, L. (2017). Storytelling for social change: Leveraging documentary and comedy for public engagement in global poverty. *Journal of Communication, 67*(5), 678–701.

Côtè, J. (1996). Sociological perspectives on identity formation: The culture–identity link and identity capital. *Journal of Adolescence, 19*(5), 417–428.

Davison, K., Jurkowski, J., Li, K., Kranz, S., & Lawson, H. (2013). A childhood obesity intervention developed by families for families: Results from a pilot study. *International Journal of Behavioral Nutrition and Physical Activity, 10*, 3. https://doi.org/10.1186/1479-5868-10-3

Duhigg, C. (2012). *The power of habit: Why we do what we do in life and business*. Random House.

Farrelly, M., Healton, C., Davis, K., Messeri, P., Hersey, J., & Haviland, M. (2002). Getting to the truth: Evaluating national tobacco countermarketing campaigns. *American Journal of Public Health, 92*(6), 901–907. https://doi.org/10.2105/ajph.92.6.901

Fox, O., & Stoett, P. (2016). Citizen participation in the UN sustainable development goals consultation process: Toward global democratic governance? *Global Governance, 22*(4), 555–573. https://www.jstor.org/stable/44861200

Freimuth, V., & Quinn, S. (2004). The contributions of health communication to eliminating health disparities. *American Journal of Public Health, 94*(12), 2053–2055. https://doi.org/10.2105/ajph.94.12.2053

Freire, P. (1970). *Pedagogy of the oppressed*. Continuum.

Garrett, L. (2015). Ebola's lesson: How the WHO mishandled the crisis. *Foreign Affairs*, September/October. https://www.foreignaffairs.com/articles/west-africa/2015-08-18/ebola-lessons?campaign=Garrett

Graybiel, A. (2008). Habits, rituals, and the evaluative brain. *Annual Review of Neuroscience, 31*, 359–387.

Green, M., & Brock, T. (2000). The role of transportation in the persuasiveness of public narratives. *Journal of Personality and Social Psychology, 79*(5), 701–721. https://doi.org/10.1037/0022-3514.79.5.701

Gustavsen, B., Hanson, A., & Qvale, T. (2008). Action research and the challenge of scope. In P. Reason & H. Bradbury (Eds.), *Handbook of action research* (2nd ed., pp. 63–76). Sage.

Habermas, J. (1987). *The theory of communicative action* (Vol. 2: Lifeworld and system: A critique of functionalist reason). Bacon Press.

Haldane, V., Chuah, F., Srivastava, A., Singh, S., Koh, G., Seng, C., & Legido-Quigley, H. (2019). Community participation in health services development, implementation, and evaluation: A systematic review of empowerment, health, community, and process outcomes. *PLoS One, 14*(5), e0216112. https://doi.org/10.1371/journal.pone.0216112

Haslam, S. (2014). Making good theory practical: Five lessons for an applied social identity approach to challenges of organizational, health, and clinical psychology. *British Journal of Social Psychology, 53*, 1–20. https://doi.org/10.1111/bjso.12061

Hecht, M. (2009). Communication theory of identity. In S. Littlejohn & K. Foss (Eds.), *Encyclopedia of communication theory* (pp. 139–141). Sage.

Hecht, M., Warren, J., Jung, J., & Krieger, J. (2004). Communication theory of identity. In W. Gudykunst (Ed.), *Theorizing about intercultural communication* (pp. 257–278). Sage.

Holtgrave, D., Wunderink, K., Vallone, D., & Healton, C. (2009). Cost-utility analysis of the national truth campaign to prevent youth smoking. *American Journal of Preventive Medicine, 36*(5), 385–388. https://doi.org/10.1016/j.amepre.2009.01.020

Johnston, H., Laraña, E., & Gusfield, J. (1994). Identities, grievances, and new social movements. In E. Laraña, H. Johnston, & J. Gusfield (Eds.), *New social movements: From ideology to identity* (pp. 3–35). Temple University Press.

Jung, E., & Hecht, M. (2004). Elaborating the communication theory of identity: Identity gaps and communication outcomes. *Communication Quarterly, 52*(3), 265–283.

Kral, M., & Allen, J. (2016). Community-based participatory action research. In A. Jason & D. Glenwick (Eds.), *Handbook of methodological approaches to community-based research: Qualitative, quantitative, and mixed methods* (pp. 253–262). Oxford University Press.

Le Bou, N., Sator, F., & Yazdi, P. (2021). *Good communication practices in community engagement*. How-to guide series of the International Federation of Red Cross and Red Crescent Societies.

Llamas, C., & Watt, D. (Eds.). (2010). *Language and identities*. Edinburgh University Press. https://www.jstor.org/stable/10.3366/j.ctv2f4vprr

Maslow, A. (1943). A theory of human motivation. *Psychological Review, 50*(4), 370–396.

Melucci, A. (1989). *Nomads of the present: Social movements and individual needs in contemporary society*. Temple University Press.

Melucci, A. (1995). *The process of collective identity*. Temple University Press.

Melucci, A. (1996). *Challenging codes: Collective action in the information age*. Cambridge University Press.

Michie, S., van Stralen, M., & West, R. (2011). The behaviour change wheel: A new method for characterising and designing behaviour change interventions. *Implementation Science, 6*, 42–79.

Murphy, S., Frank, L., Chatterjee, J., & Baezconde-Garbanati, L. (2013). Narrative versus nonnarrative: The role of identification, transportation, and emotion in reducing health disparities. *Journal of Communication, 63*(1), 116–137. https://doi.org/10.1111/jcom.12007

National Cancer Institute. (2008, June). *The role of the media in promoting and reducing tobacco use*. Tobacco control monograph no. 19. U.S. Department of Health and Human Services, National Institutes of Health, National Cancer Institute. NIH Pub. No. 07-6242.

Obregon, R., & Mosquera, M. (2005). Participatory and cultural challenges for research and practice in health communication. In H. Oscar, T. Thomas, & E. Hylland (Eds.), *Media and glocal change: Rethinking communication for development* (pp. 233–346). CLACSO.

Obregón, R., & Tufte, T. (2017). Communication, social movements, and collective action: Toward a new research agenda in communication for development and social change. *Journal of Communication, 67*(5), 635–645. https://doi.org/10.1111/jcom.12332

Obschonka, M., Silbereisen, R., Cantner, U., & Goethner, M. (2015). Entrepreneurial self-identity: Predictors and effects within the theory of planned behavior framework. *Journal of Business and Psychology, 30*(4), 773–794. https://doi.org/10.1007/s10869-014-9385-2

Paul, B. (Ed.). (1955). *Health, culture and community: Case studies of public reactions to health programs*. Russel Sage Foundation.

Polletta, F., & Jasper, J. (2001). Collective identity and social movements. *Annual Review of Sociology, 27*, 283–305.

Prakash, P. (2021, April 19). *Protocol breach blamed for second COVID case*. Fiji Broadcasting Corporation Archive. https://www.fbcnews.com.fj/news/covid-19/protocol-breach-blamed-for-second-covid-case/

Republic of Fiji. (2020). *Stakeholder engagement plan, Fiji Covid-19 emergency response project (P173903)*. Fiji Ministry of Health and Medical Services. https://www.health.gov.fj/wp-content/uploads/2020/06/Fiji-COVID-19-SEP-Final-P173903.pdf

Rise, J., Sheeran, P., & Hukkelberg, S. (2010). The role of self-identity in the theory of planned behavior: A meta-analysis. *Journal of Applied Social Psychology, 40*, 1085–1105. https://doi.org/10.1111/j.1559-1816.2010.00611.x

Savickas, M. (2002). Career construction: A developmental theory of vocational behavior. In D. Brown (Ed.), *Career choice and development* (4th ed., pp. 149–205). Jossey-Bass.

Schiavo, R. (2016). Communicating for social and behavioral change: Reflections and highlights on the IUPHE global conference in Brazil. *Journal of Communication in Healthcare, 9*(2), 71–74. https://doi.org/10.1080/17538068.2016.1207344

Simons, J. (2021). From identity to enaction: Identity behavior theory. *Frontiers in Psychology, 12*(679490). https://doi.org/10.3389/fpsyg.2021.679490

Stackpool-Moore, L. (2006). *We are one but we are many: New thinking on how communication can support HIV social movements to achieve inclusive social change*. PANOS.

Stryker, S., & Burke, P. (2000). The past, present, and future of an identity theory. *Social Psychology Quarterly, 63*(4), 284–297. https://doi.org/10.2307/2695840

Tarrant, M., Hagger, M., & Farrow, C. (2012). Promoting positive orientation towards health through social identity. In J. Jetten, C. Haslam, & S. Haslam (Eds.), *The social cure: Identity, health and well-being* (pp. 39–54). Psychology Press.

Terry, D., Hogg, M., & White, K. (1999). The theory of planned behaviour: Self-identity, social identity, and group norms. *British Journal of Social Psychology, 38*(3), 225–244. https://doi.org/10.1348/014466699164149

Thoits, P., & Virshup, L. (1997). Me's and we's: Forms and functions of social identities. In R. Ashmore & L. Jussim (Eds.), *Self and identity: Fundamental issues* (pp. 106–133). Oxford University Press.

Vallone, D., Cantrell, J., Bennett, M., Smith, A., Rath, J., Xiao, H., Greenberg, M., & Hair, E. (2018). Evidence of the impact of the truth FinishIt campaign. *Nicotine & Tobacco Research, 20*(5), 543–551. https://doi.org/10.1093/ntr/ntx119

Verplanken, B., & Faes, S. (1999). Good intentions, bad habits, and effects of forming implementation intentions on healthy eating. *European Journal of Social Psychology, 29*(5–6), 591–604.

Wallerstein, N., & Bernstein, E. (1988). Empowerment education: Freire's ideas adapted to health education. *Health Education Quarterly, 15*(4), 379–394. https://doi.org/10.1177/109019818801500402

West, R. (2007). The PRIME theory of motivation as a possible foundation for addiction treatment. In J. Henningfield, P. Santora, & J. Bickel (Eds.), *Drug addiction treatment in the 21st century: Science and policy issues* (pp. 24–34). John's Hopkins University Press.

Wiggins, N. (2012). Popular education for health promotion and community empowerment: A review of the literature. *Health Promotion International, 27*(3), 356–371. https://doi.org/10.1093/heapro/dar046

8

Hashtag Stay Healthy: Digital Media for Health Communication

Overview

If health communication decisions were solely based on whether a communication channel has vast numbers of users, then digital media and especially social media would probably be the perfect medium. The use of social media has not only grown rapidly in the past 20 years, but they have become central to more and more of our daily activities and social encounters.

As of January 2022, global internet usage has climbed to 4.95 billion (62.5% of the world's population). With more than two-thirds (67.1%) of the global population now using mobile devices, a trend expected to grow by close to 2% year-on-year, digital usage is predicted to grow increasingly mobile (GSMA Intelligence, 2022; Statista, 2022a). Hereby, social media reign supreme. Having grown by over 200% in usage between 2012 and 2022, there are now 4.62 billion social media users worldwide, equating to 58.4% of the world's population or about 75% of the world's population over 13 years of age (Kepios Analysis, 2022). As for market or user share among the competing platforms, the order depends on personal liking, absolute app download, or total usage time,

O. Werder, *Transformational Health Communication*,
https://doi.org/10.1007/978-981-99-9606-3_8

but the usual suspects lead that list. Meta's Facebook, WhatsApp, and Instagram, Google's YouTube, Tencent's WeChat, and Bytedance's TikTok are used by one to three billion users per month and are the favourite applications of one in six people globally (Data.ai, 2022; Kepios Analysis, 2022; Statista, 2022b).

Equally impressive is the average time spent using digital media, which has grown close to 7 hours daily by the end of 2021. Excluding average sleep time of 7–8 hours, people now spend more than 40% of their waking hours online. Of those, social media make up 35% of the total, or an average of 2–1/2 hours daily (GWI, 2022). While the usage varies by platform (close to 20 hours per month on Facebook vs. roughly 5 hours per month on X/formerly Twitter) as well as by country (from a high of more than 10 hours per day in South Africa to a low of 4–1/2 hours in Japan) (Data.ai, 2022; GWI, 2022), there is little doubt about the centrality of social media for our everyday lives.

Yet, we do not or ought not to choose a channel solely based on impressive general usage figures but apply a holistic view of a choice based on purpose, experience, and usability. While I do not want to give the impression of a digital media rejector, recognising a media channel's relevance and benefit might mean, in a manner of speaking, that all that glitters is not gold. To explore the relationship of health communication to information or communication technologies we start with a brief history.

A Brief History of ICT for Health

Among the earliest forms of health information and communication technologies (ICT) is most likely telehealth a.k.a. telemedicine. The idea of providing home- or community-based healthcare and consultation via telephone, and later via radio and TV/video has been experimented with since the early 1900s (Institute of Medicine, 2012). While telehealth was essentially comprised of the use of telecommunication systems to deliver healthcare remotely, by 1999 ideas to broaden the use of technology and hence make it more cost-effective led to a neologism, known as e-health (Mitchell, 2000).

The term e-health (or e-Health) was coined by the health industry to align it with the equally rising idea of e-commerce. It describes the increased ability of the combined use of electronic communication and information technologies in the health sector to perform multiple health-related functions, such as electronic data storage, transmission, and exchange (e.g., medical records), remote patient monitoring, mobile health a.k.a. mHealth (including self-care and monitoring devices used by patients or the general public for education/prevention), besides the ongoing improvement of healthcare via cyberhealth consultation and asynchronous instructions (Della Mea, 2001).

Given such a broad usage, e-health has no unifying concept, but rather contested definitions based on involved stakeholders, role of distance, and actual benefits of included technologies. With the yet non-consensual definitions of health and well-being, we discussed in earlier chapters, it is probably unsurprising that 'health' hereby is looked at primarily as a (healthcare) process, rather than an outcome. Oh et al.'s (2005) substantial review of the term's usage found that technology was viewed both as a tool to enable a process or service and "*as the embodiment of eHealth itself* (e.g., *a health website on the Internet*)." ICTs hereby play a support function to support or enrich human activities, rather than to replace them. Besides this ostensibly positive association, another thing that all reviews seemed to agree on is that e-health initiatives do not typically originate with patients or members of the public, unless those become members in patient-based tech-savvy organisations (Ball & Lillis, 2001; Oh et al., 2005; Pagliari et al., 2005; Silber, 2004).

The savvy reader may have noticed that e-health/telehealth technologies focus mostly on the treatment and management of illnesses, in short are used for applied healthcare, rather than the promotion of health. This should come as no surprise since health ICTs are usually defined as applications, devices, or databases that aim to make patient-centred care both more efficient (lower cost) and effective (improved quality). In addition, they serve to make care operations systemically more fluid, geographically flexible, and overall, less error prone (Talking Health Tech, 2020). This is not to say though that ICTs cannot aid with health promotion efforts. The fact that efforts can be personalised at low cost via ICT devices and applications that are already in regular use make them quite attractive for health promotion activities. Given that those technologies—whether they are hand-held wearable monitoring tools, stand-alone kiosks, personal computers, or social media applications—require a targeted public to actively participate in whatever the aim of the effort is, the success and wide acceptance depend on the public's willingness to manage their own health and use digital technologies as a tool to do so (Evers, 2006).

Digital Health Promotion

To discuss digital promotion of health adequately, we need to revisit the murky interpretation of what, or rather who, health promotion is for, as it certainly impacts the way we do and understand digital health promotion as well. The simple dictionary definition of 'promoting' is '*to support or actively encourage the progress or development of something*,' in our case someone's health. This indirectly says that this something exists in at least a basic way but needs some fostering. In concrete terms, health promotion is for people who are essentially healthy but need assistance in preserving this health via the promotion of lifestyles conducive to health and well-being. Aside from the previous point that modern health promotion expects a public who is actively engaged in their health (something that monitoring tools and apps are quite useful for), the question remains where we place all those digital activities primarily meant for those who have slid down the health path to ill health or imminent risk. For example, is a daily SMS reminder to diabetics to not forget their check-ups and insulin still part of health promotion, or is it part of healthcare? I don't mean to be pedantic on vocabulary definition but declaring a social media platform or website an effective tool for promotion when in fact this medium elegantly assists with treatment and care options means that we have a bit of a discrepancy. Let's start, however, with the comparably easier part of active engagement by the public.

Online Health Information-Seeking Behaviour

Along with the leap in information technology and especially web-based and social media in the last 10–20 years came the increasing popularity of proactively searching for whatever information was needed and rapidly finding something. Since most people tend to have an interest to stay healthy and understand symptoms that may endanger that desire of perfect health (see, e.g., the enduring popularity of family health books such as the Mayo Clinic's *Family Health Book* or the British Medical Association's *Complete Family Health Encyclopedia*), a quick and easy avenue like websites and posts to obtain this information was bound to become a widespread behaviour.

In the past decade, the number of US Americans, for example, who had ever searched for health information online increased from 53% to 74% (Fox & Duggan, 2013; Fox & Jones, 2009). Interestingly, the number of those who found that search easy (called '*accessing health information without frustration*') was significantly lower at around 38% (Finney Rutten et al., 2019). The number in Canada is comparable at about 69% of all Canadians (StatCan, 2021). In Europe, an average of 55% aged between 16 and 74 have sought online health information, led by the Scandinavian countries (68–77%), the Netherlands (76%), and Germany (70%) (Eurostat, 2021). In the UK, the share of people searching for health information online increased from an average of 55% in 2015 to 66% in 2020 (Statista, 2021). Numbers in Asian countries are even higher, led by Vietnam (86%), Indonesia (85%), Japan (80%), and China (79%) (Ministry of Public Management, 2015; Taira et al., 2020; Wang et al., 2021).

While these numbers are impressive, they need to be qualified by who is most likely to visit online health sites. A Pew internet research study (Fox, 2011) revealed that two groups are the most active seekers of health information online: adults who provide unpaid care for a loved one and people who face or faced a serious medical emergency. Two further interesting facts jump out. Any recent change in physical health that are not an emergency, such as weight loss, quitting smoking, or becoming pregnant, does not lead to a significant increase in online health information-seeking compared to those who did not undergo such changes. In addition, one's overall education level seems to create a significant gap in online information access, something that is studied under (digital) media literacy. This is often a result of ability (having online experience) and access (possessing broadband or other reasonably fast and secure online connections) (Fox, 2011).

On the upside, increases in searches for diet, fitness, and exercise point to an overall interest in wellness aside from medical health issues, a result that is explained with government agencies increasing their awareness messaging on these topics or existing websites being more organised and better navigable (Evers, 2006). Moreover, looking for health information online appears to have a positive effect on adhering to any suggested treatment, once the condition has been confirmed (Maon et al., 2017). However, according to a Pew Research Study (Fox & Duggan, 2013) a third of adults do not just look up information but actively engage in online self-diagnosis, i.e., use online sources to figure out on their own what their condition is, their symptoms mean, or what to do about it. Curiously, only a little over 50% then talk to a doctor about their online self-diagnosis, and about 40% find confirmation from said doctors. i.e., 50–60% of all of those who use online health information to establish their illness status and next steps either live with this online finding (and possibly self-treat it) or are being told how their 'playing doctor' has led to erroneous conclusions.

Note as well that eight in ten online health inquiries start at general search engines, punching in some keywords. Only a small minority goes straight to specialised health sites. Although some health entities, including government departments, have commenced to purchase keyword search terms and hence pop up at the start of a search engine's results list, the very fact that this is the nature of results ordering makes it clear that every information can be the first one if an entity paid for it. As a result, we cannot be too sure that whatever is seen first is indeed the best information.

Aside from concerns of people finding a potpourri of real, hyped up, and misleading information—one may recall the myriads of fake COVID cures that floated around on the Internet for example—the existence of Dr. Google and WebMD may impact a doctor-patient encounter, let alone relationship, in a detrimental fashion. The area of communication training for medical professionals both in terms of creating dialogue and trust connections has been studied for some time now (Mata et al., 2021; Omura et al., 2017). The notion that some doctors talk over patients' heads and take little time to get to know a patient has been a common finding and may explain in part the popularity of those online sites. But in the rather complex world of medicine where symptoms and causes are not singular, i.e., there is not one clear symptom for a specific disease, it often requires an actual physical examination (possibly followed by other tests and examinations) to get to the bottom of an illness and provide the most adequate treatment. Cutting out that process or demanding from one's doctor the proverbial purple pill that cures an already self-diagnosed ill is at best frustrating for the expert on the other side and at worst leads to debate and further lack of harmony and trust besides lack of cure, or worse, physical harm.

Another relevant particularity of digital health-seeking behaviour is that it typically involves (soon-to-be) patients, i.e., people who have a direct interest in restoring or maintaining a threatened state of their health. Yet, as I mentioned earlier, health promotion usually aims at maintaining good health among those who already (or still) possess it. Granted, healthy individuals may occasionally use the vast library of online health information to pursue good health or lifestyle, but they have no need to consult any doctor nor follow up on any health agency advice—digital or traditional. The biggest danger here is that the exposure to 'bad' information or being forced to make choices as a lay person based on a smorgasbord of information is very real.

The net takeaway from all this is that people do prefer the digital environment to look for health information—granted, people with a health issue more than others but still (Jia et al., 2021). So, while this information disseminating part of health promotion has always been the biggest aspect of how the run-of-the-mill health promoting agency understood their role, i.e., provide the public with sufficient information and 'how-to' self-help ideas, it has congenially transferred into the digital space to be consumed more. The core concern—and biggest job for official health-promoting services at the same time—is not being distinguishable amidst a sea of voices touting their best solution to a health issue. In short, while 'playing the digital info source' game is vital, it is equally if not more vital to be the most-trusted, liked, and loyalty-inducing source. This requires creating a reasonably close relationship with one's target groups. But this seems hard to achieve with just giving people information (a rather factual act), nor is this all we would hope a health communicator would do.

Changing Promotional Effort—The Social Media Ecology

As I laid out in the beginning of this chapter, social media have permeated our communication today. So, it is fitting to recall once more that communication in general has a factual (information dissemination) and social (relationship formation) aspect, which is why I make the 'meaning sharing' function in health communication a central tenet of this book. How then are digital media able to incorporate or even improve on both aspects, if at all? I dabbled on the first one above already.

A reasonably good working definition of the general social media characteristics has been provided by Kaplan and Haenlein (2010), who defined social media as "*a group of Internet-based applications that (…) allow the creation and exchange of user generated content.*" They highlighted a media-related and social dimension component. The former involves social media's approximation ability of face-to-face communication, affecting their capacity to reduce ambiguity and uncertainty. The latter is based on Goffman's (1959) notion of self-presentation, whereby individuals' interactions serve to engage in impression management. Granted this is not a complete overlap but one could construe the media component as the more factual aspect of communication, while the social dimension component matches quite well with communication's social function.

To date, the biggest social engagement activity is happening among people themselves in their various health-specific Facebook, Instagram, or other social media chat groups. The fact that these groups exist is a promising sign that people are open to discuss their beliefs and feelings about their health through digital media platforms. In fact, the socialising function typically takes centre stage in those groups. What is equally noteworthy though is that health experts (especially official government and medical staff) are hardly part of these groups, something that is occasionally desired by these chat groups. Plus, we ought to be reminiscent that it is again typically people with a health condition, who seek out the companionship of others with a similar burden (or their carers) as those seek and provide a more personal and realistic connection.

Equally relevant for engaging in participatory communication efforts is that those interested in using digital, and especially mobile technology to maintain or improve their health are those called high engagers in self-management. To the contrary, those who have little to no self-involvement in the management of their health not only have minimal engagement with mHealth apps but are rather sceptical about using technology as a means of self-management, calling them a burden (Desveaux et al., 2018). For example, a systematic literature review on weight loss management/healthy eating apps found that while these apps can be effective in producing weight loss through lifestyle changes in eating behaviours and physical activity patterns, their operational function (need for passive data entry), necessity of a certain level of technology and health knowledge, and the acceptability of and satisfaction with the mHealth app procedure (known as social validity) revealed a pattern where higher engagement with mHealth applications was associated with greater treatment adherence and consequent goal achievement (Dounavi & Tsoumani, 2019).

What it tells us is that successful case studies do not necessarily make a digital approach generalisable to the wider population. Undoubtedly digital media address some of the limitations in traditional health communication, namely better accessibility, interaction, engagement, empowerment, and customisation. As such, they hold considerable potential for health promotion and other health intervention activities (Levac & O'Sullivan, 2010). Notwithstanding these documented benefits and the popularity of social media, their causal impact on health, and the mechanisms through which their content influences policymakers' practice have remained unclear (Mendoza-Herrera et al., 2020; Welch et al., 2016).

A Glimpse into the Future

In 2017, PWC published an online newsletter describing the eight emerging technologies that will revolutionise business in the future (Likens, 2017). Those are Artificial Intelligence (AI), Augmented Reality (AR), Blockchain Technology, Drones, the Internet of Things (IoT), Robotics, Virtual Reality (VR), and 3-D Printing.

Deloitte Insights organised their tech trends outlook along the impact of emerging technology opportunities on 'innovation areas,' such as interaction, information, or trust, to which they then subsumed technologies that will assist with moving these areas forward (Bechtel, 2023). For instance, they foresee a move in the interaction area towards simplicity, where technologies that power human-computer interaction get more complex, but user experiences get simpler due to advancements in extended reality such as ambient experiences and neural interfaces (i.e., digital assistants monitor, and neural interfaces afford direct communication between gestures and even biological thought). Information, at the same token, moves to intelligence, which points to better and more skilled AI, including such things as affective AI (machines with personality!) and general-purpose or polymath AI, i.e., machines that can imitate a collection of human traits. While the entire report is worth a read, for our purposes we deduce a presumed growth in AI, AR/VR (here called extended reality), and decentralised platforms (which include Web 3.0 and Quantum computing).

Now, there are probably many other interesting reports and future outlooks out there that foresee one or the other digitised technology to lead the changes of the future. The main idea of picking those two—besides the fact that I consider the source reasonably credible and neutral entities—is to have some baseline to argue and explain from when we start focusing on health, and especially health communicative or promotional sources of the future. It merits remembering that the origin for health ICTs was mostly focused on improving the care aspect of health, such as doctor-patient or health system-patient interactions. So, when we come across novel tech trends, we need to be mindful what purposes they serve. For instance, VR to train new doctors or guide current ones in surgical procedures (something akin to pilot training simulators) is in my opinion not part of what we ought to focus on, when we look for tech that aids disease-prevention/health promotion. We therefore need to put aside all future health tech that has other purposes. One would logically assume that trends such as robotics, IoT, 3D printing, and drones would thus not play a major role here.

What is more promising is technology that aids with target data analysis and differentiated segmentation, followed by personalised dissemination of messages appealing to behaviour modification. As McGuire et al. (2021) have aptly noted, "*few public health campaigns have exploited the full potential that emerging technologies have to offer [and] many [government] organisations have plenty to do to reach the pinnacle of [a digitally enhanced] campaign maturity curve.*" Like many other researchers, I too have personally noticed over the years that while health(care) organisations are aware of the importance of and, in many instances, are interested in using technology for public health campaigns, a vast number of public health agencies have moved slowly to using digital tools and technologies to basically assist with their traditional strategies for public health campaigns, i.e., social media or text messages fulfil the function of disseminating the message to more or the same groups.

In other words, for many promoters it seems more important to upskill to a smart use of current technologies in the promotional communication space before entertaining adding future improvements. But ... maybe one can do both. So, let's look at how health communication may possibly look in the future.

Tomorrow's Health Campaign

Although we need to be mindful that technology has afforded competitive voices to officially designated health promotion agencies, such as local to national health departments or NGOs, to have a means to reach people, I plan to focus primarily on the health promotion professional segment here. I will add one more time that we are not interested in exploring all technology advances that happen in the health space but focus on those that have a relevance and applicability for prevention or promotional communication activities.

I remember when the Internet was 'it' back in the early 2000s everyone wanted to have a website to share information and if possible, sell their brand. E-commerce was all the rage even when a brand was quite unsuited to be sold via the Internet. As we discussed above, e-health also grew exponentially during that time, mostly via a lot of health information-sharing. Yet, Evers, 2006 report on the use of the Internet for health promotion provided a rather pessimistic view of the potential for the adoption of the Internet for health promotion programmes beyond static information sources. It concluded:

> *[while] the majority of respondents had used the Internet to get health information (80.5%), only 24.7% had used programs on the Internet for health behaviour, health promotion, or disease management [and a] majority (62%) had no intention of starting to use health-behaviour–change programs on the Internet in the foreseeable future.* (Evers, 2006, p. 6)

Although this example describes a more established (or dare we say 'old') technology, it is fitting to show that purely using the latest tech does not create a better campaign outcome. It may be unsurprising that to date the most popular social media pages and posts are not those by healthcare organisations so the substantial use of social media by the world's population is not necessarily causally linked with the idea that having a Facebook page and X/Twitter account will mean a better prevention behaviour outcome. What I discussed elsewhere applies here as well. Health promotion agencies should not solely rely on data and technology-enhanced precision in message dissemination. They need to create messages and calls-to-action that are more personalised by tailoring them to an individual's specific needs and having an empathetic understanding of the challenges they face. Once we manage to make communicative experience more inclusive and human, we can hope to move people towards a culture of wellness and prevention (Moudatsou et al., 2020). Three aspects where the effective use of technology can assist with the work show promise for the years ahead.

Improved Audience Segmentation through Big Data Analysis and AI

One of the key ideas from social marketing was to segment target audiences for messages to be more pinpointed and thus effective. Despite increased use of social media platforms, traditionally health promotion audiences are usually segmented by demographic characteristics such as age, gender, or ethnicity. What we do need—and what social marketing textbooks endorse in principle—is grouping audiences along behaviour and the statements people make about them (COVID-19 prevention or general vaccination behaviours or the lack thereof may be a good illustration why that matters). These behavioural comments happen nowhere more regularly than on people's social media accounts and groups.

Around 2005, digital communication researchers began to realise just how much data users generated through Facebook, YouTube, and other social media. Harvesting and dissecting these voluminous complex data sets, known as big data, required new data processing software but was ultimately able to address business problems that couldn't have been addressed before (OCI, 2023). What big data analysis enables an organisation to do is compile all the different data from social media, website visits, and other sources and use it to improve the communication experience, e.g., by delivering personalised messages that not only keep people interested but deal with someone's (health) issues proactively. What facilitates and will facilitate this is the growth in AI, cloud computing, and machine learning as part of the Internet of Things (IoT). For instance, one would envision a pooled data gathering from exercise and nutrition wearables, sensors, mobile devices, and smart gym equipment as part of the data for obesity prevention efforts.

What digital (big) data will provide is twofold. One, using AI affords to rapidly mine this rather unstructured vast amount of data for what issue or sub-issue is discussed at a point in time, who influences a discussion, what people are discussing, or where—digitally and geographically—a conversation happens. And two, having achieved that, they allow to identify groups on similarities in behavioural patterns and key behavioural drivers, which resolves our above idea to move towards behavioural segmentation that drive audience actions (McGuire et al., 2021).

AI-driven data collection and analysis are also good at what is known as *social listening*, a continuous social media and digital devices monitoring activity to "*track conversations and mentions related to a chosen topic on social media platforms, and then analyse them for insights into what actions you can take that will improve the experience*" (Gough, 2020). As I discuss elsewhere, a relational understanding of health communication inclusive of the histories, meanings, and evolution of social practices that impinge upon people's health and well-being efforts is important to interpret sentiments and underlying drivers of behavioural patterns of health topics discussed online. There is great promise in technology assisting effectively with pinpointing and interpreting behavioural segments and how to reach them accurately. Some published results on vaccination (Teng et al., 2022), nutrition (CDC, 2007; Montgomery et al., 2019), suicide & self-harm prevention (Calzon, 2022), or prevention of unintended pregnancy of minority teenagers (Bonnevie et al., 2021) underscore the value of this approach.

Personalised Messages and Campaigns

Having acquired better targeting segments, the logical second step is to engage those targets with more personalised messages or campaigns. We know that it is often the case that people who are the targets of traditional health promotion and behaviour change campaigns do not share the values they are being asked to adopt. If we think about campaigns intended to promote a 'healthy lifestyle,' it is important that researchers and campaigners understand the meanings this has for people and the values that are bound up with it, including their (dis)connections with meanings that are promoted in the media and health promotion campaigns, among other sites.

We would want to consider how people assess the healthiness of their current lifestyles and whether there are areas where they would like to do better and the features of their everyday lives that enable or constrain them in doing so (Lindsay, 2010). For instance, in a campaign targeting individuals who do not get their COVID booster vaccinations, the message could be tailored differently for those who are still worried about COVID as compared to those chatting about how the pandemic is all over now. One may rightfully assume that the same messaging and outreach may not resonate with both groups.

Some of the more beneficial key personalisation strategies obviously include social and communication parameters, I discuss elsewhere, such as relevant health behaviour theories, human-centred or humanistic approaches, and social practice methods. But technology will enhance those by:

1. Locating and effectively using or collaborating with culturally relevant social media influencers.
2. Utilising adaptable (via machine learning) app or wearable technology that provides contextual behavioural encouragement prompts based on feedback and current behaviour (Rabbi et al., 2015).
3. AI-based conversational tools that mimic human face-to-face interaction to overcome contact hesitancy due to the sensitive nature or stigma potential of a topic, such as mental health or sexual health (see, e.g., the "Layla's Got You" teen pregnancy prevention campaign in Bonnevie et al. (2021)).

While these examples show some effective use of AI and social media platform technology, I would concur with those (Lutkenhaus et al., 2019; McGuire et al., 2021), who say that they are tools to enhance a generally changed attitude towards audience engagement via a more community-involved approach. Using a humanistic participatory angle provides an increase in responsivity as a discussed health issue is relevant and possibly urgent to a community. The benefit of the technology lies hereby in having found the 'right' sociodemographic profile, cultural composition, or external influences of local norms on behaviour. Furthermore, community involvement can empower audiences, leading them to share perceptions and preferences, and instil an element of trust in the process (Kia-Keating et al., 2017).

Leveraging Micro-Influencers

What seems certain today is that for some groups (e.g., teenagers, young adults, cultural subgroups) online relationships developed through social networks play an increasingly important role in their lives and communication via these networks have strengthened behavioural norms and established common interests and trust. In this context, so-called influencers, individuals who influence an exceptionally large number of their peers, form standards of orientation and unless working in a collaborative or likeminded manner can undermine the best designed government health campaign (Pilgrim & Bohnet-Joschko, 2019).

Given that influencers are uniquely suited to shape perceptions and behaviours due to their established level of trust with their audiences, they can help drive greater impressions and engagement using social media (McGuire et al., 2021). Collaborating with the right influencers to amplify a campaign's message within their communities benefits public health efforts in that they can gain credibility and further engagement by those target groups. Whereas this appears all techy and social media-centric, the success of media influencers goes back to established theoretic models of social representation and social practice, where people try to make sense of the social worlds they live in and their roles in those worlds by actively negotiating and performing a wide range of practices and establishing relational values as codes for social exchange (Moscovici, 1984; Marková, 2000). Not only does this explain the weight put on suggestions brought forth by trustworthy digital 'friends' but overall underscores the relevance of a relational and representational approach to constructing health communication.

Among the host of social media influencers, the most promising group to leverage community feelings towards influencing audiences' beliefs and perceptions, and thus, future behaviour are so-called micro-influencers. These are those social media influencers, who have 10,000 to 100,000 followers and are likely to be viewed as a friend or a peer as opposed to a celebrity (online or real life) with millions of fans. While all influencer types generate greater impressions and engagement with that user-generated content (Gough et al., 2017), due to their more authentic position towards their influence group and the size of those circles, micro-influencers are better suited to reach niche groups than mass-appeal prominent individuals (Guo et al., 2020). That is, rather than selecting influencers based on their large following, to drive post impressions, further thought should be given to the influencer's social media "tone of voice" and whether the intervention messages are in line with the influencers and their following (Gough et al., 2017). Identifying the most influential users in the network and predicting the propagation of messages is where machine learning, AI, and big data analysis can assist with. As campaigns related to flu vaccine increase among minority populations in the United States (Bonnevie et al., 2020) and youth tobacco prevention (Kostygina et al., 2020) have shown, there is great potential to increase the impact of a social media campaign when working with relevant micro-influencers. This may even include non-human ones as the AI-persona called Layla in the "Layla's Got You" teen pregnancy prevention campaign has shown (Bonnevie et al., 2021).

Heal Thyself!—Being Part of Digital Health Engagements by the Lay Public

It is certainly true that various public health departments have started to increasingly use social media to reach and engage with audiences, as much as corporate entities have started to incentivise their employees to move more or use a free gym pass by providing wearables or proprietary apps or wellness-related intranet sites. But for the most part technology is used by people independently of any outside source.

For one, some more motivated or competitive individuals use apps, weblets, or other digital technology in the form of walking/fitness apps, blogs, or watch, mobile phone, or wearable fitness trackers to participate in friendly challenges and digital awards or other tokens of achievement. While some may not use them for health improvement, they are slowly changing the way we take care of ourselves and others.

Unfortunately, there are a few barriers and drawbacks. The same usage problems native to all digital technology, namely a demographic profile mismatch between heavy users vs. those most in need of 'digital contact' exists among health apps and other health tech. The costly price points of many devices are a deterrent for those that could benefit from them the most. This is compounded by design flaws, such as lack of perceived benefit by recipients when an app is overly static (e.g., most calory tracker apps offer manual entry of meals eaten only and then only deliver a daily total number), or an overly complex or annoying technology setup or repeated malfunctions (e.g., daily or hourly notifications when nothing has happened like the "you-can-still-get-your-move-goal-today" message I get in my Apple Watch when I wasn't moving enough).

Finally, as flashy and fun as many health apps and gadgets may appear, most have been designed and are run without participation of any health provider or expert. One may argue that for calorie counting or pedometer apps one only needs a tech-savvy person, but if those apps work well but do not help much in explaining my health trajectory (or lack thereof) to me, they become less engaging and probably less useful in the long run. All in all, those hands-on technologies have not been the breakthrough means to get a sizeable number or targeted individuals to engage, let alone change behaviours. More often than not, they cater to a tech-enthusiast who also happens to be fairly healthy and active.

The other broad area are social media communities, chatting with each other. I stumbled over their prevalence some years ago when I was engaged in a project on pre-diabetes/diabetes groups in the western suburbs of Sydney, Australia where we found an active group of multicultural diabetics staying in touch via WhatsApp. A few months later, a student of mine coincidentally conducted a literature review on global diabetes groups, joining and following for a short while US-based Facebook and Instagram groups. The key findings in either case were that participants were attracted to these groups because they provide what no official source does (or did), namely moral and emotional support for the "tough times" of the disease, when someone feels emotionally low or drained and needs an open and understanding ear. In addition, they offer each other tips and tricks on how to manage one's condition or answer a question, somebody did not know (e.g., whether one can still lift weights in a gym with diabetes). As you are probably aware, there are thousands of these disease-specific groups on social media platforms, either regionally, nationally, or occasionally globally, with some being open to all and others having closed formats with application options to remain more private.

Before someone wonders whether a health promoter can mimic or partake in such groups, note that the overwhelming majority are composed of people who already have a particular illness or ailment. I emphasise this again because a large portion of our promotional communication is addressed at target groups without any health condition but maybe debatable lifestyle choices. With some exceptions (e.g., drinking reduction, smoking cessation, stop depression) healthy people are not typically part of any social media health group they engage with. Can those groups exist? Possibly, but they would need an angle that attracts people from a particular behavioural segment. For example, obesity prevention cannot be about obesity prevention but maybe healthy cooking or social group activities like walking groups in the form of a friendly step or distance competition. We need to keep in mind though that it is the mutually shared pain, fear and small successes as well as having found someone who truly understands 'how I feel' that keep social media groups connected. These bonds are harder to sustain with people who may share a common interest (e.g., like to win achievement badges) but otherwise have a looser connection.

The exception is cult-like fan groups of a social media influencer as I noted above. We see those in healthy eating, exercising, body shaping, physical appearance (linked to tanning and other exposures) and social lifestyles (linked to a variety of non-communicable and even communicable disease issues from social drinking, drug experimentation (or warnings thereof) to ignoring virus protection methods that reduce one's social life (or alternatively create pro-protection alternative partying ideas). Most of these influencer-led groups have a life of their own. Whereas they may not be hostile to a potential involvement of government health agencies joining them, they are aloof if not suspicious as to those attempts. This is somewhat understandable because official health promotion services are known to typically use digital technology to give users information, which for many social media communities does not give them anything that adds value. In conclusion, since many of these groups are not competing with official sources, the net takeaway should be to collaborate in an organic way where appropriate but otherwise acknowledge their existence and possible benefit.

Conclusion

As we come to the end of this chapter, the cold hard truth is that no one will know which technology will become a circuit breaker in an often-difficult promoter-public engagement. There is absolutely no doubt that digital mobile media have become the norm for communicative interaction across ages, genders, and races, and are so ubiquitously used these days that they have become unavoidable. The point that was made here is not whether they should be used on the face of it, but whether they have been used smartly and effectively.

In the mid-1960s, the Canadian communication theorist Marshall McLuhan coined the phrase "the medium is the message" (1964). It essentially argues that the type of medium one uses influences how a message is perceived and interpreted, thus rendering the medium choice the paramount decision in a strategic or persuasive communication effort. For example, the 280-character limit on X/Twitter forces people to be to the point—avoiding unnecessary context in the process and ending up with the essence of one's communication purpose.

But as little as a hammer does not build a home, so doesn't a computer, mobile device, or algorithmic media platform communicate something by its sheer existence or popularity. They are tools that still require skilful planning and execution of one's communicative content to achieve the desired objective as did any previous delivery option. Just because you moved your smoking prevention message on an app or TikToked about COVID does not mean your message was seen, understood, or motivating.

For instance, a year or so ago I saw a state's chief medical officer rap about COVID protection on TikTok to the tunes of American rapper Popp Hunna's song Adderall (Corvette Corvette) (apparently one of the most used songs for video creations on the platform in 2022). Whereas a few people enjoyed watching it, I cannot help but question whether an artificially looking demonstration of 'I-speak-your-language' hipness was the smartest use of resources, staff, and time. In addition, 'street cred'—to stay in the jargon—needs to be earned. A top-down message listing best practice suggestions created without any input from one's target remains that whether it is delivered as spoken word in a press conference or as a sing-song rap in a short video.

That said, as the saying goes, 'you cannot not communicate,' i.e., you are always communicating no matter what delivery format. However, you may not be communicating the message you think you are. Blindly aping successful application of digital technology (or ICTs) by other industries or stakeholders is not a good approach in my opinion. Back when social marketing came onto the heath communication scene, the claim was that a social issue—like health—can be sold like a commercial brand. This was subsequently heavily debated as the context and positioning of people are different towards either topic. For instance, there is often an annoyance with the interactivity function of the social media and apps, especially among older or less tech-enthusiastic groups. To be always reachable and thus get reminders, questions or invitations on a regular basis can have a boomerang effect. As I mentioned earlier, there is at times a demographic profile mismatch of heavy user vs. those most in need of 'digital contact' and those digital health communication initiatives often lack participation by health providers or experts.

All this does not even touch upon broader tech concerns that we would now partake in as well. Those include the costs associated with tech integration and privacy issues. While the former is a moving target dependent on what one wants to do (there is quite a range from opening a free Twitter account to paying for app development to integrating AI and machine learning components into one's promotional efforts), the latter has grown in importance and is multi-faceted. There is the ongoing debate surrounding electronic records (a privacy issue onto its own) and the more sinister breaching and exploitation of private data via hacking and subsequent ransom demands (at times also automated via ransomware). Among the recent victims in Australia, for instance, was a private health insurance called Medibank where cybercriminals stole and posted on the dark web the private details, including sensitive medical information, of about 9.7 million customers. One might rightfully argue that a promotional agency will not possess such vast information of one's target groups and is hence less threatened. But we did earlier discuss the profiling of behavioural targets via AI that does include verbatim online communication of many people. And in any case most individuals do not distinguish accurately between who does what and who has access to and stored what of my information. There is a heightened sensitivity by many people to digital storage if it includes their personal information.

In the end, effective technology application in health communication and promotion will require the application of all strategic communication's decision criteria: (a) the intentionality of one's communication, (b) clear and strategic goal setting prior to message dissemination, (c) understanding of one's audience, including speaking to them in a way they will understand and appreciate, and (d) skilful analysis of post-campaign reaction.

It should be clear that this does not mean that one ought to stay away from digital and social media. To the contrary, of all that I discussed above it is evident that a smart use of, say, one's Facebook or YouTube account can enhance and improve an intervention campaign. But digital technology is not a field of dreams that magically makes things happen. The same communication skills required for traditional media and non-media communication apply. Maybe the most useful future digital technology for health communication is not the one that are easily noticed and look flashy and trendy like Twitter feeds, TikTok videos, or the latest apps. Maybe it is the one working in the background to make one's promotional planning more polished.

References

Ball, M., & Lillis, J. (2001). E-health: Transforming the physician/patient relationship. *International Journal of Medical Informatics, 61*, 1–10.

Bechtel, M. (2023). *Tech trends 2023*. Deloitte Insights. https://www2.deloitte.com/content/dam/insights/articles/us175897_tech-trends-2023/DI_tech-trends-2023.pdf

Bonnevie, E., Lloyd, T., Rosenberg, S., Williams, K., Goldbarg, J., & Smyser, J. (2021). Layla's got you: Developing a tailored contraception chatbot for black and Hispanic young women. *Health Education Journal, 80*(4), 413–424. https://doi.org/10.1177/0017896920981122

Bonnevie, E., Rosenberg, S., Kummeth, C., Goldbarg, J., Wartella, E., & Smyser, J. (2020). Using social media influencers to increase knowledge and positive attitudes toward the flu vaccine. *PLoS One, 15*(10), e0240828. https://doi.org/10.1371/journal.pone.0240828

Calzon, B. (2022, June 2). *21 examples of big data analytics in healthcare that can save people.* Business Intelligence – A datapine blog. datapine. https://www.datapine.com/blog/big-data-examples-in-healthcare/

CDC. (2007, September 20). *Segmenting audiences to promote energy balance – Resource guide for public health professionals.* Centers for Disease Control & Prevention, division of nutrition, physical activity, & obesity. https://www.in.gov/health/files/57_resource_file3.pdf

Data.ai. (2022). State of mobile 2022 report. San Francisco: Data.ai (formerly App Annie). https://www.data.ai/en/apps/unified-app/top/downloads/worldwide/overall/all-phone/?topchart=last-month

Della Mea, V. (2001). What is e-health (2): The death of telemedicine? *Journal of Medical Internet Research, 3*(2), e22. https://doi.org/10.2196/jmir.3.2.e22

Desveaux, L., Shaw, J., Saragosa, M., Soobiah, C., Marani, H., Hensel, J., Agarwal, P., Onabajo, N., Bhatia, R., & Jeffs, L. (2018). A mobile app to improve self-management of individuals with type 2 diabetes: Qualitative realist evaluation. *Journal of Medical Internet Research, 20*(3), e81–e90. https://doi.org/10.2196/jmir.8712

Dounavi, K., & Tsoumani, O. (2019). Mobile health applications in weight management: A systematic literature review. *American Journal of Preventive Medicine, 56*(6), 894–903. https://doi.org/10.1016/j.amepre.2018.12.005

Eurostat. (2021). *One in two EU citizens look for health information online.* European Union Eurostat Office. https://ec.europa.eu/eurostat/web/products-eurostat-news/-/edn-20210406-1

Evers, K. (2006). eHealth promotion: The use of the internet for health promotion. *American Journal of Health Promotion, 20*(4), S1–S7. https://doi.org/10.4278/0890-1171-20.4.1

Finney Rutten, L., Blake, K., Greenberg-Worisek, A., Allen, S., Moser, R., & Hesse, B. (2019). Online health information seeking among U.S. adults: Measuring progress toward a healthy people 2020 objective. *Public Health Reports, 134*(6), 617–625. https://doi.org/10.1177/0033354919874074

Fox, S. (2011, February 1). *Health topics: Health information is a popular pursuit online.* Pew Research Center.

Fox, S., & Duggan, M. (2013, January 15). *Health online 2013*. Pew Research Center.

Fox, S., & Jones, S. (2009, June 11). *The social life of health information*. Pew Research Center.

Goffman, E. (1959). *The presentation of self in everyday life*. Doubleday Anchor Books.

Gough, A., Hunter, R., Ajao, O., Jurek, A., McKeown, G., Hong, J., Barrett, E., Ferguson, M., McElwee, G., McCarthy, M., & Kee, F. (2017). Tweet for behavior change: Using social media for the dissemination of public health messages. *JMIR-Public Health and Surveillance, 3*(1), e14–e20. https://doi.org/10.2196/publichealth.6313

Gough, H. (2020). *Social listening: What it is and why it matters*. XM blog: Brand experience. Qualtrics. https://www.qualtrics.com/blog/social-listening/

GSMA Intelligence. (2022). *Mobile industry subscriber profile data*. Global System for Mobile Communication. https://www.gsmaintelligence.com/data/

Guo, M., Ganz, O., Cruse, B., Navarro, M., Wagner, D., Tate, B., Delahanty, J., & Benoza, G. (2020). Keeping it fresh with hip-hop teens: Promising targeting strategies for delivering public health messages to hard-to-reach audiences. *Health Promotion Practice, 21*(Suppl 1), 61S–71S. https://doi.org/10.1177/1524839919884545

GWI Worldwide. (2022). *The biggest social media trends for 2022*. GWI. https://www.gwi.com/reports/social

Institute of Medicine. (2012). *The role of Telehealth in an evolving health care environment: Workshop summary*. National Academies Press. 2012 Nov 20. 3, the evolution of telehealth: Where have we been and where are we going?

Jia, X., Pang, Y., & Liu, L. (2021). Online health information seeking behavior: A systematic review. *Healthcare (Basel, Switzerland), 9*(12), 1740–1745. https://doi.org/10.3390/healthcare9121740

Kaplan, A., & Haenlein, M. (2010). Users of the world, unite! The challenges and opportunities of social media. *Business Horizons, 53*, 59–68.

Kemp, S. (2022). *Global digital reports*. Kepios Analysis. https://datareportal.com/reports/digital-2022-global-overview-report

Kia-Keating, M., Santacrose, D., Liu, S., & Adams, J. (2017). Using community-based participatory research and human-centered design to address violence-related health disparities among Latino/a youth. *Family & Community Health, 40*(2), 160–169. https://doi.org/10.1097/FCH.0000000000000145

Kostygina, G., Tran, H., Binns, S., Szczypka, G., Emery, S., Vallone, D., & Hair, E. (2020). Boosting health campaign reach and engagement through use of social media influencers and memes. *Social Media + Society, 6*(2), 1–12. https://doi.org/10.1177/2056305120912475

Levac, J., & O'Sullivan, T. (2010). Social media and its use in health promotion. *Interdisciplinary Journal of Health Sciences, 1*(1), 47–51. https://doi.org/10.18192/riss-ijhs.v1i1.1534

Likens, S. (2017). *The essential eight building blocks*. PWC: Emerging technologies Newsletter. https://www.pwc.com/gx/en/issues/technology/essential-eight-technologies.html/

Lindsay, J. (2010). Healthy living guidelines and the disconnect with everyday life. *Critical Public Health, 20*(4), 475–487.

Lutkenhaus, R., Jansz, J., & Bouman, M. (2019). Tailoring in the digital era: Stimulating dialogues on health topics in collaboration with social media influencers. *Digital Health, 5*. https://doi.org/10.1177/2055207618821521

Maon, S., Hassan, N., & Seman, S. (2017). Online health information seeking behavior pattern. *Advanced Science Letters, 23*(11), 10582–10585.

Marková, I. (2000). Amèdèe or how to get rid of it: Social representations from a dialogical perspective. *Culture and Psychology, 6*(4), 419–460.

Mata, Á., de Azevedo, K., Braga, L., et al. (2021). Training in communication skills for self-efficacy of health professionals: A systematic review. *Human Resources for Health, 19*, 30–38. https://doi.org/10.1186/s12960-021-00574-3

McGuire, K., Krawiec, R., Malik, N., & McInerney, J. (2021, August 18). *The future of public health campaigns: Digital strategies for amplifying influence and effectiveness*. Deloitte Center for Government Insights. https://www2.deloitte.com/us/en/insights/industry/public-sector/successful-digital-public-health-campaigns.html

McLuhan, M. (1964). *Understanding media – The extensions of man*. McGraw-Hill.

Mendoza-Herrera, K., Valero-Morales, I., Ocampo-Granados, M., Reyes-Morales, H., Arce-Amarè, F., & Barquera, S. (2020). An overview of social media use in the field of public health nutrition: Benefits, scope, limitations, and a Latin American experience. *Preventing Chronic Disease, 17*, 200047. https://doi.org/10.5888/pcd17.200047

Ministry of Public Management. (2015). Information communication white paper (Part I, Chapter 2, Section 2): *Diffusion of utilization of ICT beyond age URL*. http://www.soumu.go.jp/johotsusintokei/whitepaper/ja/h27/pdf/index.html.

Mitchell, J. (2000). Increasing the cost-effectiveness of telemedicine by embracing e-health. *Journal of Telemedicine and Telecare, 6*(S1), 6–9. https://doi.org/10.1258/1357633001934500

Montgomery, K., Chester, J., Nixon, L., Levy, L., & Dorfman, L. (2019). Big data and the transformation of food and beverage marketing: Undermining efforts to reduce obesity? *Critical Public Health, 29*(1), 110–117. https://doi.org/10.1080/09581596.2017.1392483

Moscovici, S. (1984). The phenomenon of social representations. In R. Farr & S. Moscovici (Eds.), *Social representations* (pp. 3–69). Cambridge University Press.

Moudatsou, M., Stavropoulou, A., Philalithis, A., & Koukouli, S. (2020). The role of empathy in health and social care professionals. *Healthcare, 8*(1), 26–32. https://doi.org/10.3390/healthcare8010026

Oh, H., Rizo, C., Enkin, M., & Jadad, A. (2005). What is eHealth (3): A systematic review of published definitions. *Journal of Medical Internet Research, 7*(1), e1. https://doi.org/10.2196/jmir.7.1.e1

Omura, M., Maguire, J., Levett-Jones, T., & Stone, T. (2017). The effectiveness of assertiveness communication training programs for healthcare professionals and students: A systematic review. *International Journal of Nursing Studies, 76*, 120–128. https://doi.org/10.1016/j.ijnurstu.2017.09.001

Oracle Cloud Interactive – OCI. (2023). *What is big data?* Oracle Australia. https://www.oracle.com/au/big-data/what-is-big-data/

Pagliari, C., Sloan, D., Gregor, P., Sullivan, F., Detmer, D., Kahan, J., Oortwijn, W., & MacGillivray, S. (2005). What is eHealth (4): A scoping exercise to map the field. *Journal of Medical Internet Research, 7*(1), e9. https://doi.org/10.2196/jmir.7.1.e9

Pilgrim, K., & Bohnet-Joschko, S. (2019). Selling health and happiness how influencers communicate on Instagram about dieting and exercise: Mixed methods research. *BMC Public Health, 19*(1), 1054–1060. https://doi.org/10.1186/s12889-019-7387-8

Rabbi, M., Pfammatter, A., Zhang, M., Spring, B., & Choudhury, T. (2015). Automated personalized feedback for physical activity and dietary behavior change with mobile phones: A randomized controlled trial on adults. *JMIR mHealth and uHealth, 3*(2), e42. https://doi.org/10.2196/mhealth.4160

Silber, D. (2004). The case for eHealth. *Studies in Health Technology and Informatics, 100*, 3–27.

StatCan – The Daily. (2021, June 22). *Canadian Internet use survey, 2020.* Statistics Canada. https://www150.statcan.gc.ca/n1/daily-quotidien/210622/dq210622b-eng.htm

Statista. (2021). *Share of people in the United Kingdom searching health information online from 2015 to 2020, by age group*. Statista. https://www.statista.com/statistics/1245145/united-kingdom-internet-users-seeking-health-information-by-age/

Statista. (2022a). *Social media usage worldwide – Report*. Statista. https://www.statista.com/statistics/278414/number-of-worldwide-social-network-users/

Statista. (2022b). *Most popular social networks worldwide*. Statista. https://www.statista.com/statistics/272014/global-social-networks-ranked-by-number-of-users/

Taira, K., Murayama, T., Fujita, S., Ito, M., Kamide, K., & Aramaki, E. (2020). Comparing medical term usage patterns of professionals and search engine and community question answering service users in Japan: Log analysis. *Journal of Medical Internet Research, 22*(4), e13369. https://doi.org/10.2196/13369

Talking Health Tech Newsletter. (2020). *Healthcare terms: Health information and communication technologies (ICT)*. THT Pty. Ltd. https://www.talkinghealthtech.com/glossary/health-information-and-communication-technologies-ict

Teng, S., Jiang, N., & Khong, K. W. (2022). Using big data to understand the online ecology of COVID-19 vaccination hesitancy. *Humanities and social sciences. Communications, 9*(158). https://doi.org/10.1057/s41599-022-01185-6

Wang, X., Shi, J., & Kong, H. (2021). Online health information seeking: A review and meta-analysis. *Health Communication, 36*(10), 1163–1175. https://doi.org/10.1080/10410236.2020.1748829

Welch, V., Petkovic, J., Pardo Pardo, J., Rader, T., & Tugwell, P. (2016). Interactive social media interventions to promote health equity: An overview of reviews. *Health Promotion and Chronic Disease Prevention in Canada: Research, Policy and Practice, 36*(4), 63–75. https://doi.org/10.24095/hpcdp.36.4.01

9

Back to the Roots: Using Health Communication to Connect

Overview

This final chapter aims to connect all that I have discussed about health communication under the umbrella of the genuine intent of all communication. With this I hope that it leads to a rethinking of how communicating about health and prevention is practised, which would be the transformation the book carries in its title. As I mentioned in the opening chapter, the origin of the word '*communication*' contains the idea of a process of sharing or exchanging ideas, feelings, and experiences between two or more people as much as it describes an imparting information or transmitting information.

Alas, as early as 1963, PR scholar John Marston wrote: "*One of the most serious dangers in public communication is the illusion of having achieved it when in fact there has been no communication—only a one-way outpouring*" (p. 249). This quote—although not intended just for the area of public health—summarises well the reduction of communication to its contribution in strategic, often mass-mediated, marketing. This, in turn,

O. Werder, *Transformational Health Communication*,
https://doi.org/10.1007/978-981-99-9606-3_9

reduces health communication to a linear, unidirectional, expert-driven flow of information to appeal to cognitive individualistic capabilities (Lee & Garvin, 2003).

Since communication can take many forms, health communication is in principle open to a host of theories, models, and strategies and ongoing debates and critiques about best approaches and precise objectives to achieve better health. Given the centrality of language and communicative sharing in human activity, of which health is a crucial one, health communication plays a sizeable role beyond promotion and marketing discussions. It has the potential to function as a simple but relevant gateway to reduce the barriers that prevent more effective healthcare and outreach and offer a holistic idea of well-being.

In the past years, I had noticed that especially clinical therapy settings for substance abuse, addiction, and mental issues (e.g., drugs, alcohol, depression) experiment with new inclusive and participatory approaches. For example, a recent Australian Indigenous alcohol abuse centre report discussed how therapists are asked to consider not only the context of the individual within their family but also consider the context of the family in relation to the broader social, political, and historical systems. As part of the counselling, there is an emphasis on building, strengthening, and repairing relationships of the affected individual (Van de Ven et al., 2023).

These avenues to improve the communal and communicative interplay between the various stakeholders in a health communication situation—typically, the government or NGO health promoters, clinicians, or healthcare staff in general, the target individuals or groups, and then also relevant members of their social environment—form the essence of how I would define a transformation of health communication. Although talking about illness rather than health, Kleinman (1988) proposes that having honest and open discourse with people regarding their health situation helps immensely in learning about people's own version of their status, in turn assisting with prevention, cure, or palliative care. He states that "*cultural values and social relationships shape how [people] perceive and monitor [their] bodies, label and categorise bodily symptoms, [and] interpret complaints in the particular context of [their] life situation*" (p. xiii).

At the individual level, health communication ought to connect with the idea that human communication in its core is more about the sharing of meaning than the dispersion of information. As a simple thought experiment, think about whether a conversation with an acquaintance or even stranger about a mutual topic of interest (let's make it your favourite sports team) versus reading an instruction manual or listening to a lengthy lecture filled with statistics and causal arguments is more rewarding or memorable to you.

This means that a human-centred communication model in its simplest form regards communication as a dialogue between equal discourse partners. Subsequently, personal values and responsibilities, spirituality, culture, and especially self-actualisation become as relevant for a campaign plan as the usual theoretic constructs of attitudes, normative adherence, self-efficacy, and cognitive learning ability. Self-actualisation, derived from work on social representation and identity theories, is a construct that accounts for a person's (or group's) self-identity.

Our identities and the ways we see and represent ourselves shape how we communicate, what we communicate about, and how we communicate with and about others. Hence, self-awareness, pursuing goals that represent one's life mission so to speak, and choosing to be involved in resolving a challenge require communication of both the differences and commonalities (Hall, 1967; Markova, 2007) of discourse partners. It explains the discontent with the ambiguous results of employing individualistic, asocial, and acultural constructs of mainstream cognitive social psychology in messages (Moscovici, 2008), and thus might enable a sender to learn why people resist a message action item in the first place. This sort of feedback is something that a one-directional instructional statement does not ask for. Equally, to communicate to and with entire communities, one equally needs to employ a system of common understanding, in particular concepts and ideas that have meaning for that social group.

The new concepts I introduce and discuss here can, I believe, transform health communication in that they make the thinking about its process more reflective and thus more inclusive. They are not meant to replace existing practices in policy and promotion, as persuasive media campaigns and culturally sensitive policy will always be relevant. In that sense, they can be understood as complementing, if not enriching those and campaigns' pre-execution preparations at different levels. Among themselves, the concepts harmonise as well since they reside at various levels but discuss similar themes. Communicating from a position of the health humanities is an overall theoretic orientation of what health practice, care, and maintenance ought to look like. It forms the broadest perspective. It is followed by a different thinking about human health behaviour and how to address it, applying social practice theory. This mid-tier level affects campaign research and planning. On the 'lowest' or practical level we look at the procedural approaches of narrative interviewing and narrative executions as an alternative to fact and risk dissemination.

Platform: Health Humanities

For those unfamiliar with this term, health humanities are a research and practice approach that engages the arts and humanities for healthcare and well-being in a way that democratises those latter fields. At first blush, it appears to be a rival to the comparable field of medical humanities, which primarily deals with the human aspects of medicine (e.g., ethics in healthcare) to train more compassionate medical experts (see Hooker, 2008 for details). Yet, health humanities essentially aim to absorb medical humanities into other alternative approaches, such as arts and health, social prescribing, or various therapy approaches, such as music, arts, movement (Crawford, 2020). In simple terms, while medical humanities strive to move healthcare sector staff to become more insightful about the human condition, health humanities aim to include various, often overlooked, stakeholders to get involved in healthcare, prevention, and improvement.

Having multiple disciplines and groups involved in or contribute to health and well-being naturally changes its communication, which is why I find it a fitting theoretical framework for transformative health communication. As Crawford et al. (2010, 2015) explain, the equalising of the biomedical lens with non-medical public knowledge and challenge of a reductive use of the arts and humanities as a treatment option affords health humanities to "*fracture the expert to non-expert dynamic*" and shows both "*fault lines in professionally determined interventions over grassroots self-and community help*" as well as "*benefits of social and cultural assets.*"

Essentially, health humanities want patients, health service users, informal carers, and any self-caring group to get involved and co-design, co-create, or co-learn about a particular health or disease condition while living with, or having experienced, poor health because of it.

What it also means is an embrace of an interdisciplinary approach to health education and training, moving away from biomedical, often quantitative, modes of investigation and towards interpretive methods and social experiences, often leading to health activism (Charise, 2017). It is this potential for activism for public health through the arts and humanities that appears to be an asset as it demonstrates how population health improvement can be achieved without the clinically sanctioned assets. As Crawford et al. (2015) conclude, "*health humanities are a free-form and viral movement that can inform and transform ways of seeing or conceiving health care, health, and well-being*" (p. 19).

Application in Transformative Health Communication

If you believe like I do that health is and has a "societal value" (Anderson & Nishtar, 2011), then everyone ought to have an interest and stake in mutual health maintenance or improvement. Interpersonal two-way communication would play a crucial role for community dialogue and active participation. Although the shift towards a neoliberal ideology towards public health and responsibilities for one's health in the 1970s' espoused self-efficacy, self-esteem, and self-reliance from the state's citizenry, it stopped short of seeking true citizen participation and health behaviour negotiations with an engaged public. In the end, the main goal was less responsibility for all aspects of a person's health behaviour by the health system.

It is accepted that neoliberalism's move towards individual responsibility became a building block of the new public health discourse (Bacchi, 1999; Briggs, 2003; Merrild et al., 2011). Addressing health as a lifestyle problem did not just open health discourse up to the above-mentioned values debate, but also to the view that each citizen has control over her daily life, known as agency (Illsley, 1980), and needs to act accordingly.

Subsequently, health messages did become more hands-off (called nudging) but—I would argue—remained top-down 'best practice' suggestions (do this, don't do that, and here is how), which appeared to direct people's choices, and often irritated or alienated the very groups that were targeted (Whitehead & Russel, 2004). Especially policy-based interventions kept being perceived as paternalistic infringements by the message sender (usually the government). Pushbacks against mask-wearing and public place check-in directives that were in place in many countries during the height of the COVID pandemic illustrated this well. In the end, this seemingly inclusive thinking led to poorer collective health and well-being (Card & Hepburn, 2022).

Among the reasons for this result is that traditional health promotion paradigms kept assuming that any resistance (towards these new soft suggestive directives) can be overcome with smarter communication messages, well-tailored to segments of the population deemed to be non-compliant. As I illustrated in previous chapters, this neglects an understanding of why people may question expertise, normalise "unhealthy" or "risky" practices, and endorse values other than biomedical health, such as identity, belonging, pleasure, and social well-being in documenting and accounting for their health-related decisions and practices (Crawshaw & Bunton, 2009; Fox, 2002). Plus, the rather odd interpretation of free will or choice making (you are responsible for your own health, but I tell you what responsibility looks like), missed the opportunity to create a truly co-designed communication environment. To achieve the latter, policymakers would have to advance structural interventions that suggest a "we're-in-this-together" attitude rather than asking for individual-level behaviour modification when it comes to one's health. Neoliberalism may have intensified the resistance from those most in need of healthcare.

While critics may rightfully argue that marketing-based promotional efforts already cater to understanding the consumer of a communication message, this is purpose-driven rather than an attitudinal positioning. More precisely, I do not reject the notion that a purposive message—as all health communication efforts are or ought to be—benefits from a purposive approach that approximately follows a social marketing perspective. But one cannot deny that this purpose is habitually independent of the desire, let alone cooperation, of a target group. The singularity of distilling all possible beneficial knowledge about a targeted group into the "perfect" health issue message is often devoid of understanding the targeted individuals in their entirety, let alone be much concerned with their own position on the matter.

Ideas about health and what it means to be healthy are laden with values and constituted within and by different worldviews. As such, there is very likely to be a discrepancy between expected and actual message reception and response (Raphael, 2000; Stephens, 2008). The manner and circumstances in which health issues become problematised illustrate the rhetorical significance of communication of health conditions beyond the epidemiological realities as they create moral imperatives for self-management.

The way a health-humanities framework has the potential to inform health communication is through this simple attitude shift in how we look at a target individual and her social surrounding when planning a communicative effort. This may include talking to these others, like family or carers, rather than the target person herself. Overall, the new platform from which all health communication would originate would subsequently humanise the way we approach people and then engage with them communicatively.

Health communication practised under this paradigm would not stop at merely creating centrally conceived messages with a broad dissemination of its information. It would be the tool with which co-creation can occur by creating or growing relationships and trust between involved parties. In doing so, communication output, i.e., the prevention/intervention message, would become more inclusive of the histories, meanings, and evolution of social practices that impinge upon people's health and well-being efforts.

It is at this intersection where elements of agency and health resistance become a space for meaning contestations and negotiations. Like a product that is bought not for its functional value but for how it makes one feel so is a health risk message judged against its social or personal impact. It is here where communication could be used to a create a more caring world in practice but where currently professional practices and institutions conflict with this objective.

Since representations are inherently intersubjective practices, born out of dialogue and debate, such debates surrounding meaning can only be developed and re-developed within a community of others (Philogène, 2001). Health beliefs, practices, and their discourse and contestation can only occur in relationship and mutual respect. For health humanities to achieve its goal as a viral movement that transforms ways of seeing or conceiving healthcare, health, and well-being, a transformed health communication approach would be a significant tool. At the same time, health humanities provide the perfect frame, in which this communication transformation can be nurtured. In a way, the two concepts live in a symbiotic relationship.

Strategy: Social Practice Approach

While social practice theory, or shorter, practice theory is its own independent body of social theory within sociology, I find it a useful practical lens paralleling the less tangible suggestions by health humanities to activate participation in health and healthy behaviours. What it shares with health humanities is exploring and endorsing individual agency and its relationship to context, or social structures. Practice theory emerged in the late twentieth century and was first outlined in the work of the French sociologist, Pierre Bourdieu (2016).

Social practice approaches draw inspiration from a variety of theoretical traditions, most notably the aforementioned scholarship of Pierre Bourdieu (1990) but also that of Anthony Giddens (1984), whose concepts have been variously taken up by scholars seeking to overcome the divide between structure and agency in social theory. It is essentially a reaction to the Structuralist school of thought (Lèvi-Strauss, 1966) that looked at human behaviour as a consequence of existing innate universal structures. This perception would logically render human behaviours, including health behaviours, as identical across all human societies, governed by such structures.

In its attempt to make agency a vital component of creating and recreating one's social world—or assembling and reassembling the structures, in which one lives—social practice shifts the focus of inquiry away from the attitudes, discrete behaviours, and choices of individuals to socially embedded practices that are shaped by one's habitus and socialisation (Halkier, 2015). Aiming to understand relationships between agency, structure and, in our case, health, contemporary social practice theories provide an alternative, and more contextualised means, of understanding and explaining human action in relation to health and well-being (Maller, 2015).

This small treatise is inadequate to unravel the rich depth of what practice theories contribute, but it suffices to say that practices are not accounted for as being the behaviour or qualities of individual people, but people are featured as the carriers or hosts of a practice (Shove et al., 2012). Via the core practice elements (meanings, materials, and competences), individuals carry and perform practices (or cease to do so), which lead to a practice's continued existence or decline. For example, sharing a home-cooked dinner at the family table together includes equally the materials (foods, cooking equipment), competences (cooking skills, eating knowledge of specific meals), and meanings (cultural conventions and socially shared meanings of what, how, when to eat, and with whom). Besides contributing to social trends, these analyses are quite insightful to get to the bottom of behaviour fluctuations when it comes to—in this case—healthy eating and nutrition.

The recognition that practices are the outcomes of a specific "risk environment" usefully shifts the focus of analyses and interventions on public health matters to the social situations, processes, and structures in which individuals participate (Crawshaw & Bunton, 2009; Rhodes, 2009). A social practice approach avoids the study of one practice in isolation from the others with which it intersects as it is likely to be limited in its power to explain a current issue or social problem, as well as providing a limited basis on which to design for intervention and change (Maller, 2015). Hence, it is ideal for identifying the interconnections between social representations, communication contexts, and practical activity (Howarth, 2011).

Application in Transformative Health Communication

Whereas social practice approaches have yet to have a major influence on current health communication research and practices, I believe they are well-suited to health communication, where scholars have highlighted the limitations of dominant approaches to health communication campaigns, such as their focus on the individual, their ignorance of the context in which meanings are constructed and negotiated, and their cognitive orientation (Merrild et al., 2011; Stephens, 2008).

For example, the culture-centred approach to health communication, discussed earlier, recognises the importance of community, culture, and social context (Dutta-Bergman, 2005) as not only important but also as something often missing in health campaigns. Our primary interest as far as health communication is concerned lies in the potential for a social practice orientation to produce communication outputs that are inclusive of cultural or communal definitions of well-being and care and, at best, are co-created to become part of a social routine. Maller (2015), who I have cited before, fittingly summarises this:

> *Some behaviours currently labelled unhealthy, such as smoking cigarettes or drinking alcohol, do not necessarily qualify as practices in their own right. Instead, they would be considered smaller actions within more substantial and socially recognised practices such as taking a tea break, seeing a live band, or celebrating a friend's birthday. Such binary classifications also perpetuate existing, but unhelpful ideas, of what is good and bad in health, which are often overly simplistic and ignore the complexity and diversity experienced in everyday life.* (p. 61)

Recall how during the COVID-19 pandemic members of the public had been urged in many countries to adopt and comply with several preventative health measures, such as social distancing, mask-wearing and, once available, vaccination. Communicators regarded these as independent practices and thus drew upon the usual social marketing and promotions tactics and techniques to persuade audiences to not only consider the benefits of these practices to their own health but to the health of the wider community. Appeals were often made to protect the most vulnerable, such as older people and those with pre-existing health conditions. However, the extent to which diverse publics had been willing and able to comply with these health recommendations was contingent upon a range of factors, such as their perceptions of the threat, trust in those providing the recommendations (i.e., governments, media, health authorities), understanding of the basis for the recommendation, and the practicalities and cultural norms of their everyday lives.

In short, finding the right words or messages requires at a minimum paying attention to others' understanding of them. As I explained in Chap. 3, paying attention to common definitions and understandings in messages and discourse, in turn, requires a degree of empathy to the other (Riess, 2017). And recall that this conceptually draws on both self-awareness and social awareness, whereby the first term connects with the mental concept of self-identity (Tajfel, 1974) and the second term on having an in-depth understanding of societal and communal set-ups, problems, norms, and cultures (Goleman, 2006; Thorndike & Lorge, 1935). Research on the experience of social distancing during COVID in the UK, for example, found that people attempted to reconcile competing obligations, such as caring for or supporting family members or friends not in the same household during lockdown. Rather than seeing our relationships as intrinsic threats to health, communication following a practice approach highlights the importance of seeing them as resources we can draw on in collaborative practices of social containment (Long, 2020).

Understanding how meanings and practices related to health are shaped by local contexts and localised knowledge is not just relevant to avoid ineffective campaigns but also integral to ensuring that health promotion campaigns and interventions do not produce unintended and potentially harmful consequences (Broom, 2008; Guttman & Salmon, 2004). If we think about campaigns intended to promote 'healthy behaviours,' it is important that researchers and campaigners understand the meanings this has for people and the values that are bound up with it, including their (dis)connections with meanings that are promoted in the media and health promotion campaigns, among other sites.

Prior to sending a communicative appeal, we would want to consider how people assess the healthiness of their current behaviours and whether there are areas where they would like to do better and the features of their everyday lives that enable or constrain them in doing so (Lindsay, 2010). This would essentially require thinking about how to provide new combinations or replace the above-mentioned elements (materials, meanings, and competences) in existing practices to shift them in healthier directions, in addition to possibly encouraging the spread of new practices. Connecting and intervening at a fundamental level of people's routines, practices (such as exercising and eating, drinking, or engaging in preventative behaviours for infections) could be encouraged while others could be discouraged (Maller, 2015).

Doing so requires a reframing of the role and construction of communication campaigns. Social practice theories direct us to the importance of decentring the individual as the locus of change. This would suggest campaign efforts need to be adapted to consider the material and infrastructural factors that shape practices or impede shifts in those practices that are deemed to have harmful effects on a person's health and wellbeing (Evans et al., 2012).

While communication planning then necessitates a more involved or, what some might argue, cumbersome receiver interaction, the benefits outweigh the planning 'cost.' For one, unlike current planning for health campaigns that work from pre-established hypotheses, following social practice approaches provides time (e.g., via serial interviews) to allow participants to think about reasons behind their everyday actions and potential connections to their health. And two, they help researchers and communication practitioners to identify effective lines of further questioning since they can pay attention to the reactions of participants (Hitchings, 2012).

Insights obtained have the potential to assist communicators as well as policymakers and health professionals to develop more effective ways of supporting people in their everyday healthy-living attempts. In a crowded media environment where citizen-consumers are bombarded with a variety of advice, communication based on deep insights into actions and their motivational origins stand out as more relevant. This, in turn, maximises the potential for significant social and economic benefits by facilitating more efficient investments in health communication and promotion strategies.

Process: Narrative Communication to Construct Campaigns

The benefit to work in communication is the interaction one has with scholars in other human communication subfields besides the strategic and mediated communication area I have spent most of my academic career in. Those include, among others, interpersonal, group, organisational, and even nonverbal communication. Key questions that inform these subareas in particular are to comprehend how people communicate, why people communicate, with who people communicate in what way, and what effect someone's communicative efforts have on the other and why.

All of us can possibly remember conversations or simple passive reception of someone's talk as an audience member that had an impact on us. What was it about those communicative displays that made it so memorable? I speculate that it was the structure of the message or dialogue, which most likely came in the form of a narrative or included one or more stories or anecdotes to explain or reinforce a point. Whereas storytelling is often not well received in science, narratives offer increased comprehension, interest, and engagement. They "*follow a particular structure that describes the cause-and-effect relationships between events that take place over a particular time period that impact particular characters*" (Dahlstrom, 2014).

Effective communication requires more than the mere sending of information. It is too simplistic to assume that a unidirectional information campaign about a health risk and how to mitigate it will reinforce desired practices and outcomes if it seeks to change people's behaviours in isolation from understanding their conceptions of health and the "risk environments" that shape their practices (Rhodes, 2002).

Narrative health communication provides adult audiences with vivid, entertaining health stories that people readily engage with, which improves health responses of difficult-to-reach audiences (Slater & Rouner, 2002). Highly involving, personalised communications can create innovative and sustainable interventions that decrease societal divisions, promote health empowerment, and increase the attractiveness of self-management of health and illness among different target groups (e.g., Bastiaensens et al., 2015). Narrative communication, as such, has the potential to bridge the gap between developers of health promotion messages and their audiences (Greenhalgh et al., 2011).

Research has shown that for various large-scale health threats or risks publics actively construct images and stories of different sources of information and advice, and any mistrust in those sources borne out of those anecdotes is a critical factor in people's reluctance or resistance to complying with prescribed behaviours (Bangerter, 2014). People are also influenced by their own life story, i.e., their experiences of past health risks as they compare any new health warning with what they experienced during any previous health risk situations and how official warnings compared to the actual events (Holland & Blood, 2013). This includes the level of care and concern sources of public health advice are judged to exhibit (Heath & O'Hair, 2009).

For example, studies examining common traits of anti-vaccination believers have found higher levels of conspiratorial thinking, a lower tolerance to infringement on perceived personal freedom, and tendencies for confirmation bias (O'Sullivan and Durso, 1984; Stanovich et al., 2013), i.e., the recall and interpretation of information that confirms pre-existing beliefs as well as the creation of higher standards for evidence that contradicts those. Moreover, it was irrelevant that health science argues with facts and data against basically anecdotal evidence and personal accounts, opinions, and testimonies.

What this (anti-)vaccination debate made clear is that people's health-related beliefs and practices were inconsistent with the evidence, advice, and outcome expectations of health authorities. Rather than falling back on the typical explanation that the campaign failure was the result of public deficit or ignorance, we would do better to investigate how perceptions of trust and care figure in people's accounts and what communicative tropes create such trust and acceptance.

Application in Transformative Health Communication

I came across the idea of narratives first when I was studying the use of news media frames and the political process in my doctoral education. American political scientist Shanto Iyengar in his now classic examination of television's role in defining our notion of political accountability describes a storytelling frame known as the episodic frame. It is distinguished from the standard factual report, known as the thematic frame, by focusing less on analysis and context than on sensational dramas of individual perpetrators and victims. In doing so, Iyengar found, television news profoundly affects perceptions of political responsibility (Iyengar, 1991).

Although communication theorist may quibble that framing and narrative analysis are different issues—and I would concur—I see a clear parallel in their intent to create a particularly strong form of communication. Like the episodic frame in news reports, narratives in interpersonal or mediated discourse formats reduce the complexity of social or, in our case, health problems by using human stories (Zillmann, 2006). We know from past research that the human mind is better suited to process, store, and recall vivid information that comes from concrete examples (i.e., a person's story) compared with factual evidence or abstract data (Aarøe & Petersen, 2018; Boukes, 2022). Human stories help to organise people's memories and, by easing recall and functioning as availability heuristics, influence thought processes (Schmierbach & Boyle, 2020).

Health campaigns following the traditional logical-scientific communication path tend to provide abstract truths that are valid across a range of situations. For example, if an unhealthy behaviour (say smoking) has specific long-term health outcomes for a particular demographic at-risk group, then this finding holds true across all people belonging to that segment. An individual may then use these abstract truths to *generalise down* to a specific case (self, friend, acquaintance, or stranger one knows about) and ideally provide some level of predictive power regarding that specific.

Narrative communication, on the other hand, provides a specific case by, for instance, having an individual describe her health problems due to—in our example—a lifelong smoking habit. From this one case an individual can *generalise up* to infer what the general truths must be to permit such a specific to occur. In short, it is not just that using narrative executions lead to a different creative, they in fact trigger a very different sensemaking mechanism in people. While the scientific communication angle uses deductive reasoning (one deduces one's own case, or risk, from this general cause-effect relationship), narrative communication follows an inductive reasoning approach (the person's story is reflected upon for a general, and hence, own risk emanating from the cause-effect described in the case) (Strange & Leung, 1999).

Following from this, because logical-scientific communication aims to provide general truths as an outcome, the legitimacy of its message is judged on the accuracy of its claims. In contrast, since narrative communication aims to provide a reasonable depiction of individual experiences, the legitimacy of its message is judged on the authenticity of its situations (Kreiswirth, 1992). Besides the occasional undesirable side effect of inoculating the narrative against facts, even if those are accurate, narratives seem to offer intrinsic benefits in each of the four main steps of processing information: motivation and interest, allocating cognitive resources, elaboration, and transfer into long-term memory (Dahlstrom, 2014; Glaser et al., 2009).

If it were the case that people determine their health behaviours on their rational assessment of the value and utility of their action, the standard choice for message content in public health promotion, consisting of credible, science-backed facts, transposed into logical cause-effect sequences for right and wrong action would make sense. But as I illustrated in this and other chapters, people choose to ignore or re-interpret information that does not align with their own worldview or life story to minimise the effect on those. In practical terms, delivering a factual argument, e.g., reasons to get vaccinated against COVID, to a person whose social practices had led her to see a situation differently will not change that person's behaviour.

Since the value of more personalised health communication lies in the sharing of meaning of health and well-being, a storytelling approach appears to be a more effective tool to produce effective and sustainable health communication. Let me walk you through another short example. Although the COVID-19 virus had spread fast and furiously, a vast majority of people had not directly experienced it or suffered from it. Unlike a COVID survivor or first responder, who directly encountered the health effects, people unaffected by it personally had to use their own meaning-making of warnings and behaviour advice. Subsequently, health threats and facts were re-evaluated against effects on daily routines, such as financial and social restrictions or losses. In short, the same health issue received an altered narrative, which in turn affected the way health communication messages were received and responded to.

The cultural embeddedness of both deeds and discourse points to the idea that virtually all human knowledge is based on stories constructed around past experiences, and that new experiences are interpreted in terms of old stories (Howarth, 2011). Exploring the embeddedness of narratives about health within each community can help explain how communication receivers incorporate them into their ways of understanding and everyday talk and, as such, may help convert adverse reactions to health messages. Listening to the voices of lay people, who are often positioned in a passive way within health communication, policy, and science, provides a basis for developing health communication interventions that targeted groups find both easier and more motivational to follow and engage with.

There and Back Again—Concluding Thoughts

As we come to the end of the journey, I trust that one of the key tenets of 'good' communication has been fulfilled. Recall that in the opening chapter, I had highlighted that to understand human communication one must understand how people relate to one another. I have therefore attempted to pay attention throughout the chapters to keep this in mind when constructing the train of thought that ends here with the suggested approach elements.

I can fully comprehend published works that over the years suggested and discussed professional communication in strategic preparation and creative execution. After all, a recurring concern in health communication or promotion over the past decades has been that the field is just not professional enough to be effective, especially if its objectives are contested by (usually commercial) competition suggesting an opposite behaviour or course of action. While this is certainly still true for many disease-prevention efforts, I see the broader dilemma in health communication in the continuation of a unidirectional top-down form of information dissemination, often led by knowledge and methods from the biological and clinical sciences.

We also know from numerous examples and studies that expert knowledge and risk assessment are often contested or uncertain and public health messages sit alongside other ideas, sources of knowledge, and values that impact people's risk perceptions and decisions (Alaszewski, 2005; Lupton, 1999). Since individuals apply their own understanding to risk messages, their views and behaviours are not always consistent with public health advice if it conflicts with their everyday practices and concerns. In short, as I outlined in this book people's assessments of the quality and credibility of public health information are influenced by people's personal circumstances, lived experiences, values, and social networks (Holland & Blood, 2013). If nothing else, since most prevention issues rank low on people's radar messages that warn of possible future negative effects are met with indifference.

In the end, we need to ask ourselves what it is about the elements and process of communication that make it work. As a discipline communication has always integrated contrasting research paradigms to explore and explain the objective, structure, and dissemination of a communicative message and its reception and interpretation by a receiver. This included all aspects, whether it is the political, cultural, economic, symbolic, or social context of a communicative act. If we know one thing for certain, it is that as much as no one purposefully wants to be sicker, no one purposefully wants to reject or ignore all forms of communicative interaction. Yet, as much as the movie that receives the most accolades from art or film experts is not necessarily the box office hit among the public, so is the best-crafted prevention message not necessarily the one that succeeds in converting behaviour patterns. The answer to the movie exemplar alone provides some insights into what attracts people, which is why we ended this chapter with the storytelling design.

There are by now a few examples in health promotion where campaigns focus on narratives of individuals or slice-of-life vignettes showing common social practices and how those interact with healthy or unhealthy behaviours. In short, there are encouraging signs of experimentations with the formats I had suggested above. In the Australian context, where I work, this includes smoking cessation campaigns for both the general, e.g., the '*Never Give Up Giving Up*' campaign (Quit Victoria, 2013) and

Indigenous, e.g., the '*Don't make smokes your story*' (Australian Department of Health, 2016) publics as well as alcohol prevention aimed at parents' influencer role, e.g., the '*Kids Absorb Your Drinking*' (Drinkwise, 2008), to name a few. However, those campaigns are still outnumbered by more traditional approaches.

What fascinates me in studying communication in general holds also true for health communication, namely understanding the intricacies of human communication. I fully acknowledge critics' concern that conducting health campaigns in the fashion I propose is cumbersome and unscientific, but besides the continued muted effectiveness of current efforts, the fact that something is difficult does not make it unworthy of trial. I fully believe that complementing social marketing, education, or information campaigns with rounds of actively listening, openness to other ideas, and solicitation of input can generate insights that—if translated well into message content—can help people gain more self-awareness and formulate compelling arguments by themselves regarding their future health-related behaviours. In that sense, my call for more human-focused communication research and practice echoes Kleinman's (1988) call for better support of medical social science to deal more appropriately with illnesses:

> *Until anthropological, sociological, psychological, historical, ethical, and literary studies (the human sciences of medicine) become a substantial division of medical research, we will lack the knowledge needed to more systematically conceptualize illness experience and meanings. As long as we lack such knowledge, the development of new paradigms of practice and effective treatment strategies will be delayed, and the research enterprise will remain enormously unbalanced toward disease questions.* (p. 266)

Translating the sharing of meaning idea of communication through discussing the meanings of health we each have, the fears and barriers we see in making a change, and the steps we prefer to balance health with other important or cherished aspects of our lives, may transform health communication to a tool that can assist with better voluntary engagement, finding fulfilment in working and conversing with one another, and ultimately arriving at good health, well-being, and happiness for all in an egalitarian and democratic manner. But it does require that effort. As Hippocrates said in his treatise on ancient medicine, "*[I]f you miss being understood by laymen, and fail to put your hearers in this condition, you will miss reality.*"

References

Aarøe, L., & Petersen, M. (2018). Cognitive biases and communication strength in social networks: The case of episodic frames. *British Journal of Political Science, 50*(4), 1–21.

Alaszewski, A. (2005). Risk communication: Identifying the importance of social context. *Health, Risk & Society, 7*(2), 101–105.

Anderson, P., & Nishtar, S. (2011). Communicating the non-communicable. *Journal of Health Communication: International Perspectives, 16*(s2), 6–12.

Australian Department of Health. (2016). *Don't make smokes your story*. Australian Government Department of Health. https://www.health.gov.au/our-work/dont-make-smokes-your-story?language=en

Bacchi, C. (1999). *Women, policy, and politics: The construction of policy problems*. Sage.

Bangerter, A. (2014). Investigating and rebuilding public trust in preparation for the next pandemic [Editorial]. *European Psychologist, 19*(1), 1–3. https://doi.org/10.1027/1016-9040/a000173.

Bastiaensens, S., Vandebosch, H., Poels, K., Van Cleemput, K., DeSmet, A., & De Bourdeaudhuij, I. (2015). 'Can I afford to help?' How affordances of communication modalities guide bystanders' helping intentions towards harassment on social network sites. *Behaviour & Information Technology, 34*(4), 425–435. https://doi.org/10.1080/0144929X.2014.983979

Boukes, M. (2022). Episodic and thematic framing effects on the attribution of responsibility: The effects of personalized and contextualized news on perceptions of individual and political responsibility for causing the economic crisis. *The International Journal of Press/Politics, 27*(2), 374–395. https://doi.org/10.1177/1940161220985241

Bourdieu, P. (1990). *The logic of practice*. Stanford University Press.

Bourdieu, P. (2016). Habitus. In J. Hillier & E. Rooksby (Eds.), *Habitus: A sense of place* (2nd ed., pp. 43–52). Routledge.

Briggs, C. (2003). Why nation-states and journalists can't teach people to be healthy: Power and pragmatic miscalculation in public discourses on health. *Medical Anthropology Quarterly, 17*(2), 287–321.

Broom, D. (2008). Hazardous good intentions? Unintended consequences of the project of prevention. *Health Sociology Review, 17*(2), 129–140.

Card, K., & Hepburn, K. (2022). Is neoliberalism killing us? A cross sectional study of the impact of neoliberal beliefs on health and social wellbeing in the midst of the COVID-19 pandemic. International Journal of Health Services: *Planning, Administration, Evaluation*. Advance online publication. https://doi.org/10.1177/002073142134040

Charise, A. (2017). Site, sector, scope: Mapping the epistemological landscape of health humanities. *Journal of Medical Humanities, 38*, 431–444.

Crawford, P. (2020). Global health humanities and the rise of creative public health. In P. Crawford, B. Brown, & A. Charise (Eds.), *The Routledge companion to health humanities* (pp. 1–9). Routledge.

Crawford, P., Brown, B., Baker, C., Tischler, V., & Abrams, B. (2015). *Health humanities*. Palgrave.

Crawford, P., Brown, B., Tischler, V., & Baker, C. (2010). Health humanities: The future of medical humanities? *Mental Health Review Journal, 15*(3), 4–10.

Crawshaw, P., & Bunton, R. (2009). Logics of practice in the 'risk environment'. *Health, Risk & Society, 11*(3), 269–282.

Dahlstrom, M. (2014). Using narratives and storytelling to communicate science with nonexpert audiences. *Proceedings of the National Academy of Sciences of the United States of America, 111*(Suppl 4), 13614–13620. https://doi.org/10.1073/pnas.1320645111

Drinkwise Australia. (2008). *Parental influence campaigns*. Drinkwise. https://drinkwise.org.au/our-work/parents-campaign/#

Dutta-Bergman, M. (2005). Theory and practice in health communication campaigns: A critical interrogation. *Health Communication, 18*(2), 103–122.

Evans, D., McMeekin, A., & Southerton, D. (2012). Sustainable consumption, behaviour change policies and theories of practice. *COLLeGIUM: Studies across Disciplines in the Humanities and Social Sciences, 12*, 113–129.

Fox, N. (2002). What a 'risky' body can do: Why people's health choices are not all based in evidence. *Health Education Journal, 61*(2), 166–179.

Giddens, A. (1984). *The constitution of society: Outline of the theory of structuration*. Polity Press.

Glaser, M., Garsoffky, B., & Schwan, S. (2009). Narrative-based learning: Possible benefits and problems. *European Journal of Communication Research, 34*(4), 429–447.

Goleman, D. (2006). *Social intelligence: The new science of human relationships*. Bantam Books.

Greenhalgh, T., Collard, A., Campbell-Richards, D., Vijayaraghavan, S., Malik, F., Morris, J., & Claydon, A. (2011). Storylines of self-management: Narratives of people with diabetes from a multiethnic inner-city population. *Journal of Health Services Research & Policy, 16*(1), 37–43. https://doi.org/10.1258/jhsrp.2010.009160

Guttman, N., & Salmon, C. (2004). Guilt, fear and knowledge gaps: Ethical issues in public health communication interventions. *Bioethics, 18*(6), 531–552.

Halkier, B. (2015). Mundane science use in a practice theoretical perspective: Different understandings of the relations between citizen-consumers and public communication initiatives build on scientific claims. *Public Understanding of Science, 26*(1), 40–54.

Hall, S. (1967). *Representation: Cultural representations and signifying practices.* Sage.

Heath, R., & O'Hair, H.(2009). The significance of crisis in risk communication. In Heath, R., & O'Hair, H. (Eds.), *Handbook of risk and crisis communication* (pp. 5–31). New York: Taylor and Francis Group.

Hitchings, R. (2012). People can talk about their practices. *Area, 44*(1), 61–67. https://doi.org/10.1111/j.1475-4762.2011.01060.x.

Holland, K., & Blood, R. (2013). Public responses and reflexivity during the swine flu pandemic in Australia. *Journalism Studies, 14*(4), 523–538.

Hooker, C. (2008). The medical humanities - A brief introduction. *Australian Family Physician, 37*(5), 369–370.

Howarth, C. (2011). Representations, identity, and resistance in communication. In D. Hook, B. Franks, & M. Bauer (Eds.), *The social psychology of communication* (pp. 153–168). Palgrave Macmillan.

Illsley, R. (1980). *Professional and public health: Sociology in health and medicine.* Nuffield Provincial Hospital Trust.

Iyengar, S. (1991). *Is anyone responsible?: How television frames political issues.* University of Chicago Press. https://doi.org/10.7208/chicago/9780226388533.001.0001

Kleinman, A. (1988). *The illness narratives: Suffering, healing and the human condition.* Basic Books.

Kreiswirth, M. (1992). Trusting the tale: The narrativist turn in the human sciences. *New Literary History, 23*(3), 629–657. https://doi.org/10.2307/469223.

Lee, G., & Garvin, T. (2003). Moving from information transfer to information exchange in health and health care. *Social Science & Medicine, 56*, 449–464.

Lèvi-Strauss, C. (1966). *The savage mind.* University of Chicago Press.

Lindsay, J. (2010). Healthy living guidelines and the disconnect with everyday life. *Critical Public Health, 20*(4), 475–487.

Long, N. (2020). From social distancing to social containment: Reimagining sociality for the coronavirus pandemic. *Medical Anthropology Theory, 7*(2), 247–260.

Lupton, D. (Ed.). (1999). *Risk and sociocultural theory: New directions and perspectives*. Cambridge University Press. https://doi.org/10.1017/CBO9780511520778

Maller, C. (2015). Understanding health through social practices: Performance and materiality in everyday life. *Sociology of Health and Illness, 37*, 52–66. https://doi.org/10.1111/1467-9566.12178

Markova, I. (2007). Social identities and social representations: How are they related? In G. Moloney & I. Walker (Eds.), *Social representations and identity: Content, process and power* (pp. 215–236). Palgrave Macmillan.

Marston, J. (1963). *The nature of public relations*. McGraw-Hill.

Merrild, C., Andersen, R., Risør, M., & Vedsted, P. (2011). Resisting "reason": A comparative anthropological study of social differences and resistance toward health promotion and illness prevention in Denmark. *Medical Anthropology Quarterly, 31*(2), 218–236.

Moscovici, S. 2008 [1961]. *Psychoanalysis: Its image and its public*. Polity Press.

O'Sullivan, C., & Durso, F. (1984). Effect of schema-incongruent information on memory for stereotypical attributes. *Journal of Personality and Social Psychology, 47*(1), 55–70. https://doi.org/10.1037/0022-3514.47.1.55.

Philogéne, G. (2001). A Theory of Methods. In Deaux, K. and Philogene, G. (Eds) *Representations of the Social.* Oxford: Blackwell Publishers.

Quit Victoria. (2013). *Quit creates positive campaign*. Vic Health. http://www3.health.vic.gov.au/news/quit.htm

Raphael, D. (2000). The question of evidence in health promotion. *Health Promotion International, 15*(4), 355–367.

Rhodes, T. (2002). The 'risk environment': A framework for understanding and reducing drug-related harm. *International Journal of Drug Policy, 13*(2), 85–94. https://doi.org/10.1016/S0955-3959(02)00007-5.

Rhodes, T. (2009). Risk environments and drug harms: A social science of harm. *International Journal of Drug Policy, 20*, 193–201.

Riess, H. (2017). The science of empathy. *Journal of Patient Experience, 4*(2), 74–77.

Schmierbach, M., & Boyle, M. (2020). Concrete examples of abstract others: Testing exemplar availability as an additional explanation for third-person perceptions. *International Journal of Public Opinion Research, 32*(3), 510–529.

Shove, E., Pantzar, M., & Watson, M. (2012). *The dynamics of social practice: Everyday life and how it changes*. Sage.

Slater, M., & Rouner, D. (2002). Entertainment; education and elaboration likelihood: Understanding the processing of narrative persuasion. *Communication Theory, 12*(2), 173–191. https://doi.org/10.1111/j.1468-2885.2002.tb00265.x

Stanovich, K., West, R., & Toplak, M. (2013). Myside bias, rational thinking, and intelligence. *Current Directions in Psychological Science, 22*(4), 259–264. https://doi.org/10.1177/0963721413480174.

Stephens, C. (2008). *Health promotion: A psychosocial approach*. Open University Press.

Strange, J., & Leung, C. (1999). How anecdotal accounts in news and in fiction can influence judgments of a social problem's urgency, causes, and cures. *Personality and Social Psychology Bulletin, 25*(4), 436–449.

Tajfel, H. (1974). Social identity and intergroup behaviour. *Social Science Information, 13*(2), 65–93.

Thorndike, E., & Lorge, I. (1935). The influence of relevance and belonging. *Journal of Experimental Psychology, 18*, 574–584.

Van de Ven, K., Ritter, A., & Cunningham, E. (2023, April 25). Treatment for drug and alcohol misuse should involve families and communities. *The Conversation*. https://theconversation.com/treatment-for-drug-and-alcohol-misuse-should-involve-families-and-communities-197536

Whitehead, D., & Russel, G. (2004). How effective are health education programmes–resistance, reactance, rationality and risk? *International Journal of Nursing Studies, 41*, 163–172.

Zillmann, D. (2006). Exemplification effects in the promotion of safety and health. *Journal of Communication, 56*, S221–S237.

Index[1]

[1] Note: Page numbers followed by 'n' refer to notes.

O. Werder, *Transformational Health Communication*,
https://doi.org/10.1007/978-981-99-9606-3

C

D

SPRINGER NATURE

GPSR Compliance

The European Union's (EU) General Product Safety Regulation (GPSR) is a set of rules that requires consumer products to be safe and our obligations to ensure this.

If you have any concerns about our products, you can contact us on ProductSafety@springernature.com

In case Publisher is established outside the EU, the EU authorized representative is:

Springer Nature Customer Service Center GmbH
Europaplatz 3
69115 Heidelberg, Germany